Ultrasound-Guided Procedures

Guest Editor

HISHAM TCHELEPI, MD

ULTRASOUND CLINICS

www.ultrasound.theclinics.com

January 2009 • Volume 4 • Number 1

SAUNDERS an imprint of ELSEVIER, Inc.

W.B. SAUNDERS COMPANY
A Division of Elsevier Inc.

1600 John F. Kennedy Boulevard • Suite 1800 • Philadelphia, Pennsylvania 19103-2899

http://www.theclinics.com

ULTRASOUND CLINICS Volume 4, Number 1
January 2009 ISSN 1556-858X, ISBN-13: 978-1-4160-6365-0, ISBN-10: 1-4160-6365-X

Editor: Barton Dudlick
Developmental Editor: Theresa Collier

Ultrasound Clinics (ISSN 1556-858X) is published quarterly by W.B. Saunders, 360 Park Avenue South, New York, NY 10010-1710. Months of publication are January, April, July, and October. Business and editorial offices: 1600 John F. Kennedy Boulevard, Suite 1800, Philadelphia, Pennsylvania 19103-2899. Accounting and circulation offices: 6277 Sea Harbor Drive, Orlando, FL 32887-4800. Periodicals postage paid at New York NY, and additional mailing offices. Subscription prices are $189 per year for (US individuals), $274 per year for (US institutions), $94 per year for (US students and residents), $215 per year for (Canadian individuals), $306 per year for (Canadian institutions), $229 per year for (international individuals), $306 per year for (international institutions), and $114 per year for (Canadian and foreign students/residents). To receive student/resident rate, orders must be accompanied by name of affiliated institution, date of term, and the signature of program/residency coordinator on institution letterhead. Orders will be billed at individual rate until proof of status is received. Foreign air speed delivery is included in all Clinics subscription prices. All prices are subject to change without notice. **POSTMASTER:** Send address changes to *Ultrasound Clinics*, Elsevier Periodicals Customer Service, 11830 Westline Industrial Drive, St. Louis, MO 63146. **Customer Service: 1-800-654-2452 (US). From outside the United States, call 1-314-453-7041. Fax: 1-314-453-5170. E-mail: JournalsCustomerService-usa@ elsevier.com (for print support) or JournalsOnlineSupport-usa@elsevier.com (for online support).**

Reprints: For copies of 100 or more, of articles in this publication, please contact the Commercial Reprints Department, Elsevier Inc., 360 Park Avenue South, New York, NY 10010-1710. Tel.: (+1) 212-633-3812; Fax: (+1) 212-462-1935; E-mail: reprints@elsevier.com.

Printed and bound by CPI Group (UK) Ltd, Croydon, CR0 4YY

Transferred to Digital Print 2011

Contributors

GUEST EDITOR

HISHAM TCHELEPI, MD
Assistant Professor of Radiology, Director
of Ultrasound, Department of Radiology, Wake
Forest University School of Medicine,
Winston-Salem, North Carolina

AUTHORS

DAVID D. CHILDS, MD
Assistant Professor, Department of Radiology,
Wake Forest University School of Medicine,
Wake Forest University Baptist Medical
Center, Winston-Salem, North Carolina

WUI K. CHONG, MBBS, MRCP, FRCR
Department of Radiology, University of
North Carolina Hospitals, University of
North Carolina, Chapel Hill, North Carolina

HOLLINS P. CLARK, MD
Assistant Professor, Department of Radiology,
Wake Forest University School of Medicine,
Winston-Salem, North Carolina

EDWARD G. GRANT, MD
Professor of Radiology and Chairman,
Department of Radiology, University
of Southern California Keck School of
Medicine, USC University Hospital, Los
Angeles, California

SHANNON M. GULLA, MD
Clinical Instructor, Department of Radiology,
Wake Forest University School of Medicine,
Medical Center Boulevard, Winston-Salem,
North Carolina

ALEXANDER S. JUNG, MD
Assistant Professor of Radiology, Department
of Radiology, University of Southern California
Keck School of Medicine, USC University
Hospital, Los Angeles, California

YUEH Z. LEE, MD, PhD
Department of Radiology, University of
North Carolina Hospitals, University
of North Carolina, Chapel Hill,
North Carolina

JULIEANNE McGREGOR, MD
Department of Nephrology and Hypertension,
University of North Carolina Kidney Center,
University of North Carolina School of
Medicine, Chapel Hill, North Carolina

JOHN P. McGAHAN, MD
Vice Chair and Director of Abdominal Imaging,
Professor, Department of Radiology, University
of California, Davis Medical Center,
Sacramento, California

WAYNE MONSKY, MD, PhD
Assistant Professor, Department of Radiology,
University of California, Davis Medical Center,
Sacramento, California

**CAROL L. PHILLIPS, BSc, MBBS, MRCS,
FRCSC**
Specialist Registrar in Radiology, Department
of Clinical Imaging, Royal Devon and Exeter
NHS Foundation Trust, Exeter, Devon,
United Kingdom

BRENT T. STEADMAN, MD, PhD
Resident, Department of Radiology, Wake
Forest University School of Medicine,
Winston-Salem, North Carolina

HISHAM TCHELEPI, MD
Assistant Professor of Radiology, Director of Ultrasound, Department of Radiology, Wake Forest University School of Medicine, Winston-Salem, North Carolina

ANTHONY F. WATKINSON, BSc, MSc (oxon), MBBS, FRCS, FRCR
Professor of Radiology, Department of Clinical Imaging, Royal Devon and Exeter NHS Foundation Trust, Exeter, Devon, United Kingdom; The Peninsula Medical School, Exeter, United Kingdom

PETRA L. WILLIAMS, BSc, MBBS, MRCP
Specialist Registrar in Radiology, Department of Clinical Imaging, Royal Devon and Exeter NHS Foundation Trust, Exeter, Devon, United Kingdom

Contents

Preface   ix

Hisham Tchelepi

**Ultrasound Interventions in the Neck with Emphasis on Postthyroidectomy
Papillary Carcinoma**   1

Alexander S. Jung and Edward G. Grant

> This article reviews the sonographic technique for a basic ultrasound of the thyroid
> and a typical postthyroidectomy surveillance scan. Diagnostic criteria for these
> scans are discussed. Ultrasound-guided biopsy of thyroid nodules is reviewed, as
> are techniques for biopsy of recurrent nodal disease or disease in the thyroid bed.
> Ultrasound-guided ablation techniques are described as they apply to patients
> who have undergone prior thyroidectomy.

Ultrasound-guided Biopsies of Peripleural Lung Lesions   17

Shannon M. Gulla, Hisham Tchelepi, Brent T. Stedman, and Hollins P. Clark

> Ultrasound is an alternative to the traditional CT-guidance most often used for lung
> biopsies. Although not appropriate for all thoracic biopsies, this technique can be
> a safe and effective choice for peripleural lung lesions. As emerging technologies,
> such as image fusion, gain wider acceptance, ultrasound-guided thoracic biopsy
> will be more than a footnote. This article reviews the advantages and disadvantages
> of ultrasoundguided biopsy for peripleural lung lesions, describes appropriate tech-
> nique, and briefly discusses management of complications.

Ultrasound and Abdominal Intervention: New Luster on an Old Gem   25

David D. Childs and Hisham Tchelepi

> Ultrasound is a valuable tool for both diagnostic and therapeutic percutaneous ap-
> plications in the abdomen. Numerous advantages over CT include faster procedure
> times, real-time needle visualization, decreased cost, and a lack of ionizing radiation.
> Newer technology, such as image fusion, has allowed the radiologist to simulta-
> neously use the advantages of two modalities, ultrasound and CT or MR imaging,
> to localize lesions. Because regulatory bodies in the United States are becoming
> more aware of the risks of radiation exposure to the population from CT, ultrasound
> will regain its position as the first diagnostic imaging modality, and may become the
> imaging modality of choice for all interventions.

Ultrasound-Guided Kidney Biopsies   45

Yueh Z. Lee, JulieAnne McGregor, and Wui K. Chong

> Sonography is an excellent modality for guidance of renal biopsy. Ultrasound can
> detect potential pitfalls, direct proper placement of the needle, and identify compli-
> cations. Interventional radiology or surgical support should be available in the event
> of complications.

Ultrasound-Guided Radiofrequency Ablation Within the Abdomen   57

John P. McGahan and Wayne Monsky

Ultrasound alone can be used to guide treatment of many hepatic tumors. In the kidney, combination of ultrasound and CT is often used. Ultrasound may be used for needle placement, whereas CT is used to identify vital structures that may overlie the treated lesion, such as the ureter or adjacent bowel. Several different technical factors must be mastered before performing radiofrequency ablation in the abdomen to minimize complications and maximize results.

Pelvic Drainage: Image Guidance and Technique   73

Carol L. Phillips, Petra L. Williams, and Anthony F. Watkinson

Management of pelvic abscesses and collections can be challenging in terms of their localization and subsequent access for purposes of aspiration or drainage. Although formerly the territory of surgeons, improvements in imaging technology and applied techniques now enable interventional radiologists to perform percutaneous or endocavitary drainage of even the most difficult abscesses. Various combinations of imaging modality and route of access can be used depending on the location of the abscess, individual patient constraints, and operator preference. This article focuses on the different ultrasound-guided techniques used for pelvic drainage, including difficult access, and, equally important, discusses when it is not appropriate.

Index   83

Ultrasound Clinics

FORTHCOMING ISSUES

April 2009

Selected Topics

July 2009

Advanced in Ultrasound
Vikram S. Dogra, MD, *Guest Editor*

RECENT ISSUES

October 2009

Advanced Obstetrical Ultrasound: Fetal Brain,
spine, and Limb Abnormalities
Noam Lazebnik, MD, and Roee Lazebnik, MD,
Guest Editors

July 2008

Women's Imaging
Vikram S. Dogra, MD, and Deniz Akata, MD,
Guest Editors

THE CLINICS ARE NOW AVAILABLE ONLINE!

Access your subscription at:
www.theclinics.com

GOAL STATEMENT

The goal of the *Ultrasound Clinics* is to keep practicing radiologists and radiology residents up to date with current clinical practice in ultrasound by providing timely articles reviewing the state of the art in patient care.

ACCREDITATION

The *Ultrasound Clinics* is planned and implemented in accordance with the Essential Areas and Policies of the Accreditation Council for Continuing Medical Education (ACCME) through the joint sponsorship of the University of Virginia School of Medicine and Elsevier. The University of Virginia School of Medicine is accredited by the ACCME to provide continuing medical education for physicians.

The University of Virginia School of Medicine designates this educational activity for a maximum of 15 *AMA PRA Category 1 Credits*™ for each issue, 60 credits per year. Physicians should only claim credit commensurate with the extent of their participation in the activity.

The American Medical Association has determined that physicians not licensed in the US who participate in this CME activity are eligible for a maximum of 15 *AMA PRA Category 1 Credits*™ for each issue, 60 credits per year.

Credit can be earned by reading the text material, taking the CME examination online at http://www.theclinics.com/home/cme, and completing the evaluation. After taking the test, you will be required to review any and all incorrect answers. Following completion of the test and evaluation, your credit will be awarded and you may print your certificate.

FACULTY DISCLOSURE/CONFLICT OF INTEREST

The University of Virginia School of Medicine, as an ACCME accredited provider, endorses and strives to comply with the Accreditation Council for Continuing Medical Education (ACCME) Standards of Commercial Support, Commonwealth of Virginia statutes, University of Virginia policies and procedures, and associated federal and private regulations and guidelines on the need for disclosure and monitoring of proprietary and financial interests that may affect the scientific integrity and balance of content delivered in continuing medical education activities under our auspices.

The University of Virginia School of Medicine requires that all CME activities accredited through this institution be developed independently and be scientifically rigorous, balanced and objective in the presentation/discussion of its content, theories and practices.

All authors/editors participating in an accredited CME activity are expected to disclose to the readers relevant financial relationships with commercial entities occurring within the past 12 months (such as grants or research support, employee, consultant, stock holder, member of speakers bureau, etc.). The University of Virginia School of Medicine will employ appropriate mechanisms to resolve potential conflicts of interest to maintain the standards of fair and balanced education to the reader. Questions about specific strategies can be directed to the Office of Continuing Medical Education, University of Virginia School of Medicine, Charlottesville, Virginia.

The faculty and staff of the University of Virginia Office of Continuing Medical Education have no financial affiliations to disclose.

The authors/editors listed below have identified no professional or financial affiliations for themselves or their spouse/partner:
Matthew J. Bassignani, MD (Test Author); David D. Childs, MD; Wui K. Chong, MBBS, MRCP, FRCR; Barton Dudlick (Acquisitions Editor); Edward G. Grant, MD; Alexander S. Jung, MD; Yueh Z. Lee, MD, PhD; JulieAnne McGregor, MD; John P. McGahan, MD; Wayne Monsky, MD, PhD; Carol L. Phillips, BSc, MBBS, MRCS, FRCSC; Brent T. Stedman, MD, PhD; Hisham Tchelepi, MD (Guest Editor); and Petra L. Williams, BSc, MBBS, MRCP.

The authors/editors listed below have identified the following professional or financial affiliations for themselves or their spouse/partner:
Hollins P. Clark, MD is an industry funded research/investigator for Boston Scientific.
Shannon M. Gulla, MD owns stock in Schering-Plough.
Anthony F. Watkinson, BCc, MSc(oxon), MBBS, FRCS, FRCR serves on the Advisory Board for Biocompatibles UK.

Disclosure of Discussion of Non-FDA Approved Uses for Pharmaceutical Products and/or Medical Devices.
The University of Virginia School of Medicine, as an ACCME provider, requires that all faculty presenters identify and disclose any off-label uses for pharmaceutical and medical device products. The University of Virginia School of Medicine recommends that each physician fully review all the available data on new products or procedures prior to clinical use.

TO ENROLL

To enroll in the Ultrasound Clinics Continuing Medical Education program, call customer service at 1-800-654-2452 or visit us online at www.theclinics.com/home/cme. The CME program is available to subscribers for an additional fee of $205.00.

Preface

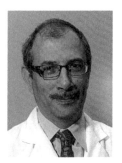

Hisham Tchelepi, MD
Guest Editor

This issue of *Ultrasound Clinics* addresses the role of ultrasound imaging-guided procedures. Despite advances in CT and MR imaging, ultrasound boasts the advantage of continuous uninterrupted real-time needle visualization, lack of radiation, and cost effectiveness. Emerging ultrasound technologies, such as high resolution linear probes, better depict a wide spectrum of abnormalities now, even at depth of 8–10cm. These probes are particularly useful for liver and kidney transplant biopsies, adding greater detail and higher accuracy.

Our goal is to present the expanding role of interventional sonography in the chest, abdomen, and pelvis, outlining the indications, techniques, potential pitfalls and complications. In addition, we will highlight exciting innovations, such as fusion imaging, a technology that melds images obtained by CT or MR imaging with sonograms. It has proven particularly valuable for biopsy procedures targeting ill-defined or small lesions.

I was fortunate to have exceptional individuals, who are experts in their fields, to contribute to this issue. I am very grateful to them. Without their dedication and hard work, this project would never have materialized. I would like to express my appreciation to my friend and colleague, Dr. David DiSantis, for his advice and support. I am also thankful to Elsevier, and specifically Barton Dudlick, for inviting me to participate. I hope you will find this issue of *Ultrasound Clinics* a useful resource in your day-to-day practice.

Hisham Tchelepi, MD
Department of Radiologic Sciences
Wake-Forest University School of Medicine
1st Floor, Reynolds Tower
Winston-Salem, NC 27157, USA

E-mail address:
htchelep@wfubmc.edu

Ultrasound Clin 4 (2009) ix
doi:10.1016/j.cult.2009.06.001

Ultrasound Interventions in the Neck with Emphasis on Postthyroidectomy Papillary Carcinoma

Alexander S. Jung, MD, Edward G. Grant, MD*

KEYWORDS

- Thyroid • Ultrasound
- Fine needle biopsy • Thyroid carcinoma
- Metastatic papillary carcinoma of the thyroid
- Cervical lymph node

Ultrasound has been the mainstay in imaging of the thyroid for many years. The superficial location of the gland makes it an ideal target for sonographic evaluation, and high-resolution images can be obtained in almost every patient. Although ultrasound can be used to examine the thyroid for various reasons, it is most commonly used to evaluate patients suspected of having a thyroid nodule and is highly accurate in this regard. Given the high incidence of thyroid nodules in the general population[1,2] and lack of specificity of the ultrasound examination with regard to their being benign or malignant,[3] ultrasound-guided fine needle aspiration (FNA) biopsy also has become a commonly performed procedure. Ultrasound-guided FNA has replaced nonguided biopsy in almost all institutions. FNA is a relatively simple procedure with minimal discomfort, few complications, and a high level of accuracy in differentiating benign from malignant nodules in experienced hands.[4–6]

Patients diagnosed with thyroid carcinoma almost invariably undergo a complete thyroidectomy with or without attendant lymph node dissection, depending on whether abnormal or suspicious lymph nodes are identified on presurgical imaging.[7–9] Patients who have undergone a thyroidectomy require postoperative surveillance, which generally includes conducting a physical examination, measuring serum thyroglobulin levels, and performing some form of cross-sectional imaging such as CT, MRI, or ultrasound. Although CT and, more recently, MR represent attractive techniques for follow-up after thyroidectomy,[10,11] ultrasound is being used increasingly for surveillance and may well represent the best modality for this task.[12] Ultrasound also has the ability to provide guidance for FNA of suspicious nodes or potential recurrent disease in the thyroid bed.[13–15] Recently, ultrasound-guided alcohol ablation of metastatic nodes has shown promise and may provide a means of avoiding repeat surgical procedures in patients who have undergone multiple prior surgeries and radiation treatment in areas of the neck.[16] Ultrasound surveillance of the postthyroidectomy neck is so sensitive in its ability to detect small-volume tumor recurrence that it exceeds our understanding of the clinical import of detecting occult residual or recurrent disease in what is usually a relatively indolent and nonaggressive malignancy.[17] Only future epidemiologic studies will indicate the true value of identifying and treating small intrathyroidal malignancies and equally small foci of recurrence.

This article reviews the sonographic technique for a basic ultrasound of the thyroid and a typical

Department of Radiology, University of Southern California Keck School of Medicine, USC University Hospital, 1500 San Pablo Street, Los Angeles, CA 90033, USA
* Corresponding author.
E-mail address: edgrant@usc.edu (E.G. Grant).

Ultrasound Clin 4 (2009) 1–16
doi:10.1016/j.cult.2009.03.001

postthyroidectomy surveillance scan. Diagnostic criteria for these scans are discussed. Ultrasound-guided biopsy of thyroid nodules is reviewed, as are techniques for biopsy of recurrent nodal disease or disease in the thyroid bed. Ultrasound-guided ablation techniques are described as they apply to patients who have undergone prior thyroidectomy.

TECHNICAL ASPECTS OF THE ULTRASOUND EXAMINATION

The thyroid gland, jugular venous lymph node chains, and most other structures in the anterior neck represent ideal targets for ultrasound imaging. Most patients can be imaged with high-frequency transducers using broadband technology, with frequencies as high as 15 to 17 MHz applicable in thin patients. In patients with particularly thick necks, lower frequency transducers may be necessary to image the more posterior portions of the thyroid gland. Optimally, Gray scale and color Doppler should be included in the examination and linear array transducers used in all patients.

During the examination, a patient typically lies in a supine position with the neck comfortably extended. The neck is optimally exposed by not having a pillow under the patient's head. In obese patients or patients with a short, thick neck, a pillow placed beneath the shoulders may hyperextend the neck and facilitate the examination. Evaluation of the thyroid should include standard transverse and longitudinal images of both lobes of the gland and the isthmus. Measurements of the lobes themselves and any identified nodules should be obtained in three dimensions. The jugular/carotid regions should be evaluated for adenopathy or other extrathyroidal masses, and the scan should proceed from the clavicle to the submandibular region. Lymph nodes should be identified and their position documented in relation to the surrounding structures; they should be measured in three dimensions for follow-up. We strongly recommend that an anatomic ultrasound worksheet be filled out by the person performing the scan in all patients; it is essential in patients undergoing postthyroidectomy surveillance ultrasound. Typically this latter group of patients is followed on a routine basis, and the ability to review an worksheet greatly facilitates this task (**Fig. 1**). At our institution we scan the worksheet directly into our picture archiving and communication system at the completion of the scan so that it is available to the technologist and radiologist when patients return.

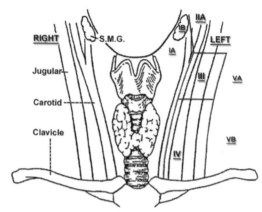

Fig. 1. Thyroid/lymph node worksheet. Technologist's worksheet that may be used for basic ultrasound examination of the thyroid or postoperative surveillance. On the patient's left, we have superimposed the node levels in red over the image to facilitate consistency in reporting, communication of node location to surgeon, and identification on future examinations. These worksheets are incorporated into the patient's examination as they are scanned into the picture archiving and communication system at the time of the study.

NORMAL ANATOMY

The normal thyroid is divided into the right and left lobes, and the isthmus is draped over the trachea in the lower neck. The normal thyroid should be homogeneous throughout and relatively hyperechoic with a variable number of vessels, which are generally most prominent at the upper and lower poles. The inferior and superior thyroid arteries and veins are often visualized in these regions. Veins may be relatively large and can be differentiated from small cysts by scanning in orthogonal planes or applying color Doppler. The right and left lobes of the gland typically lie between the carotid arteries and the trachea, with the jugular veins located somewhat laterally. The jugular veins are easily compressed by the transducer in most normal patients, which often renders them invisible. The air within the trachea typically causes intense posterior shadowing and obscures anything behind it.

Although most of the esophagus is thus rendered invisible, it is frequently visualized as a multilayered rounded structure posteromedial to the left lobe of the thyroid. Occasionally a patient's esophagus is visualized on the right as well. Although this structure is usually easily recognizable, scanning in the orthogonal plane can confirm that the rounded structure in question represents the esophagus. Patients may be asked to swallow, in which case air generally is seen passing through the lumen. Anterior to the thyroid, one typically finds the strap muscles; somewhat laterally one finds the sternocleidomastoid muscles. The triangular and hypoechoic longus coli muscles lie posterior to the thyroid and should be symmetric. The size of the normal gland is variable, but most authorities recognize a normal gland as ranging between 4 and 5 cm long and having transverse and anteroposterior dimensions less than 2 cm.

THYROID CANCER

Statistically, most (approximately 90%) thyroid malignancies are classified as differentiated cancers, the most common of which is papillary carcinoma.[8,18] Less frequently, follicular and Hürthle cell neoplasms may be encountered. They present a diagnostic challenge on FNA because differentiation between benign and malignant follicular and Hürthle cell lesions is not possible.[19] Nondifferentiated forms of thyroid cancer typically include medullary and anaplastic carcinomas, both of which tend to be more aggressive than the differentiated cancers and often present in more advanced stages. Perhaps most importantly from an imaging standpoint is the fact that the pattern of metastatic disease is different among these two groups, with differentiated cancers typically recurring locally in the form of nodal disease and undifferentiated cancers spreading to distant locations. Because of this predilection for local recurrence among the common, differentiated cancers, surveillance with ultrasound is effective.

Most thyroid malignancies are discovered by virtue of a palpable nodule found by a patient or on clinical examination. Given the frequency of neck imaging for abnormalities unrelated to thyroid disease (eg, carotid sonography, positron emission tomography, MRI/CT of the cervical spine), an increasing number of thyroid nodules are being discovered incidentally. Thyroid nodules are common in the general population, being identified in as many as 5% of women and 1% of men by palpation.[1,2] Using ultrasound, an estimated 19% to 67% of the population are found to have nodules.[20] The incidence of thyroid nodules increases with age and is higher in women, but most thyroid nodules are benign, with an approximate 5% to 10% incidence of malignancy.[21,22] Approximately 23,500 cases of differentiated cancer are diagnosed each year,[23] and the number seems to be rising,[24] likely based on a more aggressive approach to biopsy and follow-up of incidentally discovered nodules.

Given the number of nodules present in the overall population, which nodules deserve follow-up and which deserve biopsy has tremendous implications and remains somewhat controversial. Several recent consensus articles on this subject seemed to agree that nodules larger than 1 to 2 cm should be biopsied.[25–27] At our institution, we consider 1 cm to be a reasonable threshold. The selection of nodules for biopsy is complicated by the frequent presence of multiple nodules in an individual patient, and no simple guidelines are available in this common situation. Although older medical dogma suggested that patients with solitary nodules have a higher incidence of carcinoma,[28] it is relatively well established that the incidence of malignancy is equivalent in patients with multiple versus solitary lesions,[29–31] leaving us with the dilemma of which among multiple nodules to biopsy. Most authorities recommend biopsy of a "dominant nodule" in patients with multiple masses, but exactly what a dominant nodule is remains to be defined and is often a subjective decision. In addition to size, the advent of high-resolution ultrasound allows characterization of nodules. Specific features may dictate a more or less aggressive stance with regard to biopsy and—in some patients—biopsy of multiple nodules in one sitting.

Most authorities first classify thyroid nodules according to their internal echo characteristics, with lesions being classified as hypoechoic, hyperechoic, isoechoic, or mixed, cystic, and solid (**Fig. 2**A–D). Among these types, most would consider hypoechoic nodules to have the highest association with malignancy. They are also the most common, and even in this group, most are benign.[31–33] Hyperechoic lesions are also common, and although they have a lower incidence of malignancy, cancers may be found in this group. Mixed lesions are common, and as a general rule, the more cystic a lesion is, the more likely it is to be benign.[27,34,35] Unfortunately, in rare instances, malignancy may be found in largely cystic lesions and only true cysts can be confidently classified as benign. Cystic areas within solid nodules are usually secondary to liquefactive degeneration or hemorrhage within an otherwise solid nodule.

These anechoic areas may contain a variety of unrelated materials (**Fig. 3**A–C). Aspiration may produce thin, brownish material that likely represents old blood, clear serous fluid, or thick gel-like colloid that may be difficult to draw up into the needle. Unfortunately, all of these cystic lesions are particularly prone to produce a non-diagnostic aspirate because cells may be difficult to obtain. In performing an aspiration of a mixed

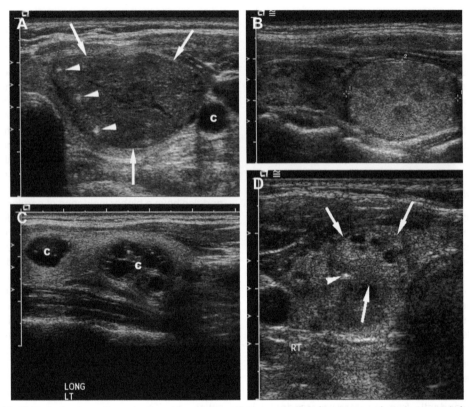

Fig. 2. (*A–D*) Typical echopatterns in thyroid nodules. (*A*) Large, well-defined hypoechoic lesion in left lobe of gland. Several echogenic foci likely representing calcifications are present posteromedially (*arrows*). FNA was diagnostic of a follicular neoplasm that was benign at surgery. (*B*) Well-defined, relatively hyperechoic nodule (*cursors*) in a multinodular gland. As the dominant nodule, it was biopsied; cytologic results indicated that it was papillary carcinoma. (*C*) Mixed cystic and solid nodules. Larger, inferior nodule is approximately 50% solid versus cystic. Note echogenic foci that have no or weak comet-tail artifact. Biopsy produced clear, highly viscous material; cytologic evaluation was consistent with a benign colloid nodule. (*D*) Isoechoic nodule with single clump-like calcification (*arrow*). Biopsy was diagnostic of a benign colloid nodule.

lesion, one should direct the needle tip to the solid components of a nodule rather than simply attempting to aspirate fluid. Some patients may experience symptomatic relief by aspirating a large amount of fluid, and such maneuvers are reasonable; however, fluid often reaccumulates over a relatively short period of time. Lesions that contain thick, viscous material are particularly frustrating and difficult to aspirate. If, on the first pass, the needle is clearly within a lesion and nothing is returned after lengthy period of suction, moving to a larger needle (usually 22 gauge) may allow aspiration of a small amount of fluid. In an effort to bias the cytologist, we usually tell them the nature of the aspirate if a lesion is largely anechoic.

Aside from the overall echo characteristics of the nodules, additional features of benign or malignant lesions should be sought. Among these, internal echogenic foci are probably the most important. Small, discrete echogenic foci are particularly worrisome because they may represent the psammomatous calcifications of papillary carcinoma. Clump-like and peripheral, so-called "eggshell calcifications" may be encountered. In the past, such patterns of calcifications were typically equated with benign nodules.[36] Although these calcifications are far less strongly associated with malignancy than punctate calcifications, increasing experience suggests that the incidence of cancer is significant. In our experience, any calcification should suggest biopsy.[37–39] On the opposite side of the spectrum, echogenic foci may be encountered that demonstrate strong, comet-tail, or reverberration artifacts. In largely cystic lesions, they may be safely assumed to be benign and representative of colloid.[40] Typically these lesions yield the clear, viscous fluid that is difficult to aspirate. Unfortunately, in our experience, the definitive differentiation between psammomatous calcification and punctate echogenic foci with weaker posterior, comet-tail artifacts

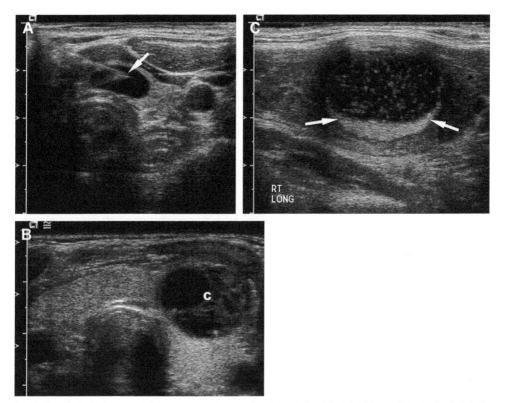

Fig. 3. (*A–C*) Anechoic lesions: colloid cyst versus hemorrhagic nodule. (*A*) Palpable nodule in the left isthmus of the thyroid is largely anechoic, although in other sections papillary projections were present. Note biopsy needle in the center of the nodule (*arrow*). Aspirate using a 22-gauge needle yielded a tiny amount of clear, yellowish, viscous liquid. Diagnosis was a colloid cyst. (*B*) Mixed cystic and solid nodule at the junction of the isthmus and the left lobe of the thyroid. Patient described rapid enlargement clinically. Although large parts of the lesion are also anechoic, aspirate in this case yielded thin, dark, reddish-brown material that was easily aspirated and consistent with old blood. Cytologic evaluation was benign colloid nodule with hemorrhage. (*C*) Large anechoic lesion in right thyroid with swirling, punctate echogenic foci typical of colloid granules. Note posterior layering (*arrows*). Aspiration yielded clear, thin material. Lesion was easily aspirated and essentially completely collapsed at the end of the procedure. Cytologic diagnosis was benign colloid cyst.

may be difficult in solid lesions and biopsy is necessary in most cases (**Fig. 4**A–D).

Other sonographic features that have been described as suggestive of malignant nodules include poorly defined or lobulated margins and nodules that are taller than they are wide.[35] Although this latter feature has been well documented in breast cancer and malignant lymph nodes, for example, it remains questionable when applied to thyroid nodules.[41] The sonographic halo sign (a hypoechoic rim around a more hyperechoic center) also has been described as being suggestive of benign disease.[42] We believe that this is of no diagnostic value and may be seen in benign and malignant lesions. Several authors have evaluated value of color Doppler in the differentiation of benign and malignant lesions (**Fig. 5**); results have been controversial.[31,43,44] As a general rule, there seems to be a higher incidence of malignancy in

hypervascular lesions. Practically speaking, size is clearly the main factor that dictates biopsy in most patients; however, other factors (described previously) may prompt biopsy in smaller lesions or suggest biopsy of multiple nodules in the same patient. Among these factors, punctate, echogenic foci are probably the most compelling. We have obtained positive biopsy results in such cases in several lesions smaller than 1 cm.

ULTRASOUND-GUIDED BIOPSY OF THYROID NODULES

Before performing a FNA biopsy, we explain the procedure to patients in detail and obtain written informed consent. The procedure is safe with theoretical complications, including bleeding, infection, and puncture of surrounding structures. In our facility, the procedure is not performed under completely sterile conditions, but we have

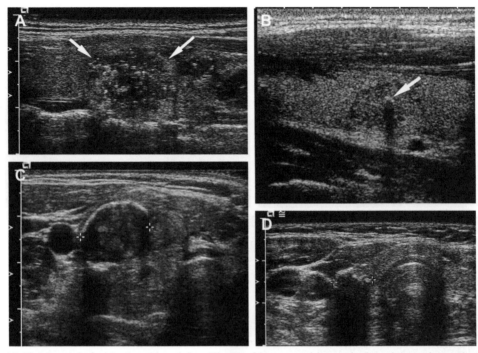

Fig. 4. (A–D) Echogenic foci in thyroid nodules. (A) Mixed hyper- and hypoechoic nodule with poorly defined borders (arrows). Note numerous punctate echogenic foci typical of psammomatous calcifications of papillary carcinoma. Comparing these to echogenic foci in Fig. 2C, one would have difficulty determining whether clear comet-tail artifacts are present in both, a common problem in solid or partially solid nodules. Cytology was diagnostic of papillary carcinoma. (B) Isoechoic lesion containing a central clumped calcification (arrow). Clumped calcifications often exhibit posterior acoustic shadowing; psammomatous calcifications do not because they are too small. Cytology was diagnostic of a benign colloid nodule. (C) Hypoechoic nodule with classic "eggshell" calcifications (cursors). Although less ominous than punctate calcifications, such lesions are still associated with an increased incidence of carcinoma and should be biopsied. Cytology demonstrated papillary carcinoma. (D) Right thyroid nodule with densely shadowing calcifications (cursors). Such nodules may be difficult to penetrate and roll away from the needle when approached. Shadowing poses additional problem of inability to clearly see needle tip until it emerges through opposite side of nodule. Cytology was diagnostic of papillary carcinoma.

yet to encounter a postbiopsy infection, and this issue is likely more theoretical than real. Bleeding is a rare but definite possibility and should be suspected upon visible swelling after puncture; ultrasound can be used to document its presence. The patient's head should be elevated and pressure applied. Unless bleeding is of sufficient magnitude to compromise the patient's airway (a complication we have never encountered), the patient can be treated conservatively and sent home once the swelling has stabilized.

Puncture of surrounding structures is possible, and lesions are often in the immediate proximity of the carotid artery and jugular veins. We have never encountered a complication secondary to puncture of the carotid artery. Although puncture of the jugular vein is avoided, venous structures can be safely traversed if necessary and light pressure applied afterwards. Accidental puncture of the trachea can occur and, in our experience, is more likely in thin patients who have undergone

prior thyroidectomy. In these patients, one may have to pass the biopsy needle close to the trachea and there is no intervening thyroid tissue. Tracheal puncture has likely occurred if there is a sudden degradation of the ultrasound image as air leaks into the soft tissues. Patients typically experience coughing and hemoptysis. These are self-limiting complications, and assurance for patients and the radiologist is all that is necessary.

Before performing a biopsy one should review any existing scans, and the physician performing the biopsy should survey the neck. Unfortunately, it is not uncommon for patients to be referred for biopsy with misleading or incorrect results from prior scans. Although explaining to patients that there is no need for biopsy may be embarrassing, most patients are relieved and grateful for the personal care. Once the lesion to be biopsied is identified, a mark is placed on the patient's skin immediately medial to the transducer. Because the jugular and carotid vessels lie lateral to the

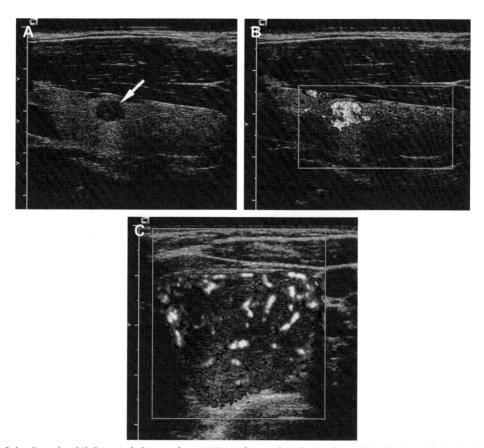

Fig. 5. Color Doppler. (*A*) Gray scale image shows a 7-mm hypoechoic lesion (*arrow*) in the thyroid gland of a local endocrinologist. (*B*) Color Doppler demonstrated intense hypervascularity. Although lesion was relatively small, biopsy was undertaken and the diagnosis was papillary carcinoma. (*C*) Large hypoechoic lesion with possible "spoke and wheel" appearance of intense peripheral vascularity and radiating pattern of internal vessels. Although this appearance was originally thought to be diagnostic of follicular lesions, this is no longer believed to be the case. Color patterns can be subjective on ultrasound, and care must be taken not to overstate their diagnostic performance. Biopsy showed this to be a Hürthle cell lesion, which was benign when hemithyroidectomy was performed.

thyroid, puncture is almost always performed in a medial to lateral orientation (**Fig. 6**). Because of the limited space between the chin and clavicle, ultrasound-guided procedures are almost always performed in a transverse orientation. It may be beneficial to place a pillow beneath the patient's shoulders (not under the neck) to provide better access in patients with short necks or large breasts. The region around the mark can be sterilized with an antiseptic agent such as povidone-iodine and a small amount of local anesthetic instilled. Although some physicians perform biopsy without anesthesia, claiming that the instillation of local is more painful than the puncture itself, we believe using local anesthesia is the best approach when multiple punctures are performed. Although local anesthesia numbs the puncture site, one should keep in mind that many patients experience pain on passing the needle through

the surface of the thyroid and one should avoid traversing this area multiple times as the biopsy needle is being moved up and down.

Before biopsy, we place the transducer in a commercially available sheath. We typically perform the biopsy with a 25-gauge needle and make three passes. A drop of the aspirate is placed on one slide and a smear is made by dragging a second slide over it. Too much material on a slide obscures detail and should be avoided. The slide should be placed in fixative immediately to prevent air-drying artifact. If available, the slides should be evaluated with a microscope before allowing patients to leave to ascertain whether a sufficient quantity of cellular material has been obtained. Most cytologists strongly recommend that fixative be drawn into the needle and syringe to wash out any adherent cellular material. Any excess liquid that is not used for slides can be

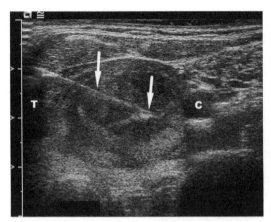

Fig. 6. Needle orientation for left lobe biopsy. Large, hypoechoic left lobe lesion with a hyperechoic "halo" lies medial to the carotid artery (C) and lateral to the trachea (T). Jugular vein is largely compressed by transducer pressure. Note approach of needle from medial to lateral anterior to trachea. Most biopsies are performed using this approach to avoid traversing vessels. Right lobe lesions would be approached from the opposite vantage point, also across trachea. One should make every attempt to monitor needle tip to avoid puncture of vessels or trachea. Cytologic evaluation showed papillary carcinoma with abundant Hürthle cells.

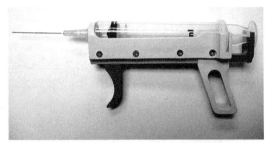

Fig. 7. Biopsy apparatus. A 10-mL syringe with a 25-gauge needle is inserted into commercially available plastic biopsy apparatus. Approximately 1 cc of air is drawn into the syringe to facilitate extrusion of the sample. "Gun-like" construction of the syringe holder allows ease of application of suction and excellent control of the needle while the radiologist's opposite hand holds the transducer and monitors position of the needle tip at all times.

placed into the fixative. This material is spun down and a "cell button" is made, which is evaluated along with the rest of the slides. In cases in which a large amount of fluid is obtained from nodules, our cytologists recommend that we send the fluid itself. Aspirated liquid typically forms a thick coagulum when placed in fixative, which may be difficult to process.

There are two schools of thought with regard to performing the biopsy itself. Some prefer aspiration of the lesion while applying suction, whereas others prefer to use the capillary action of the needle and do not apply suction. We strongly prefer the former approach. For this to be easily accomplished, the syringe should be placed in a suction gun apparatus (Fig. 7), which allows sufficient pressure to be applied to the syringe with one hand while the opposite hand holds the transducer and monitors the position of the needle tip at all times. Trying to apply pressure to the syringe itself with one hand is, in our opinion, unwieldy. For physicians who prefer the capillary technique, the needle itself is passed into the lesion under direct ultrasound guidance and moved up and down, allowing capillary action to draw material into the needle. Most would attach a syringe to the needle before removing it. In either case, one should try to ascertain that the needle is moving up and down within the nodule, rather than the

nodule moving with the needle as may sometimes be the case with hard lesions. Hard or calcified lesions may be challenging because of their propensity to move out of the way as puncture is being performed. A small amount of air should be brought into the syringe before aspiration or attachment to facilitate extrusion of the sample. One also should not lose sight of the fact that biopsy results are only as good as the cytologist reviewing the slides, and biopsy is not advisable if excellent cytologic interpretation is not available.

Biopsy results are typically divided into five categories. A diagnosis of malignancy typically dictates total thyroidectomy because thyroid cancer may be multifocal (Figs. 8 and 9).[45] Benign lesions are often diagnosed in the form of colloid nodules, and patients may be followed over time and undergo repeat biopsy if significant change in the

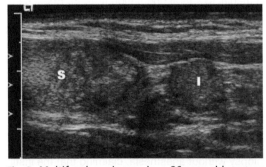

Fig. 8. Multifocal carcinoma in a 26-year-old woman with recent appearance of right thyroid nodule. Ultrasound revealed two discrete solid nodules, the more superior of which (S) was relatively hyperechoic, whereas the more inferior (I) was hypoechoic. Each was biopsied; both were diagnosed as papillary carcinomas.

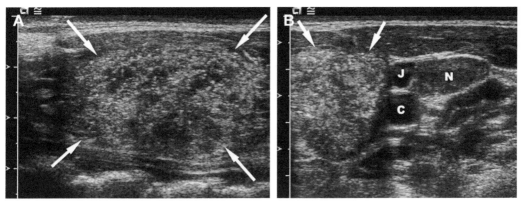

Fig. 9. (A, B) A 22-year-old woman with a large neck mass. (A) Longitudinal section through the left thyroid reveals a large nodule that occupied almost the entire lobe (*arrows*). Note innumerable punctate echogenic foci, suggesting calcifications. (B) Transverse image shows the primary mass (*arrows*) with punctate calcifications in the thyroid. Lateral to the thyroid lie the carotid artery (C) and jugular vein (J). Lateral to these vessels, multiple enlarged lymph nodes (N) were identified, which suggested metastatic disease. Biopsy confirmed papillary carcinoma. Patient underwent thyroidectomy and lymph node dissection.

lesion occurs. Although unlikely, it is possible that a sampling error could result in a false-negative biopsy result.[46] Follicular or Hürthle cell neoplasms may be diagnosed cytologically, but it is not possible to differentiate between the benign and malignant forms of these lesions without excision and gross examination of the margins of the lesion. In such cases, because the incidence of malignancy is said to be approximately 20%,[47] most surgeons perform a hemi-thyroidectomy and a separate completion procedure only if histologic evaluation is positive for malignancy.[48] Others perform a total thyroidectomy to avoid a second surgical procedure.

Occasionally, the results of biopsy may be considered suspicious or indeterminate, in which case a repeat biopsy is usually indicated. Finally, nondiagnostic biopsy secondary to insufficient material may occur. The incidence of this result should be relatively uncommon, but reports range between 15% and 20% even in experienced hands.[49] A nondiagnostic biopsy result should suggest a repeat biopsy because these lesions have a higher incidence of malignancy than the general population.[50,51] Cystic or highly vascular lesions are particularly prone to nondiagnostic results. In the case of the former, fluid may fail to yield sufficient cells for diagnosis. Lesions that contain viscous colloid are particularly problematic in this regard because it is often difficult to aspirate even a small quantity of this material. Hypervascular lesions are problematic because blood may be sucked into the aspirating syringe rather than cellular material. Advocates of the non-suction technique claim particular success in these cases, but we remain dubious. Although

core biopsy of the thyroid has been described, we have avoided this procedure at our institution in favor of repeat FNA and have had excellent results.[52] We occasionally perform FNA in patients on warfarin or aspirin and have not encountered complications, although this situation is best avoided if possible.

POSTTHYROIDECTOMY ULTRASOUND

Differentiated carcinomas are by far the most common malignancies to affect the thyroid. The typical mode of spread is to the local lymph nodes, which are easily accessible to ultrasound examination. An evaluation of the surrounding lymph nodes should be included in all patients with suspicious nodules because 20% to 30% have malignant adenopathy at the time of presentation (**Fig. 9A, B**).[53] Identification of adenopathy is essential and significantly changes treatment because lymph node dissection is undertaken in

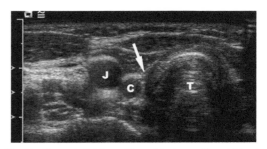

Fig. 10. Normal right postthyroidectomy thyroid bed. No intervening tissue (*arrow*) is identified between the trachea (T) and common carotid artery (C). Jugular vein (J) lies lateral to the common carotid.

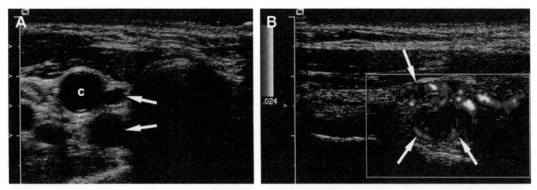

Fig. 11. (*A, B*) Recurrent disease in the thyroid bed. (*A*) Transverse section through right thyroid bed shows two discrete hypoechoic nodules (*arrows*) that were not identified on previous studies. (*B*) Longitudinal power Doppler image confirms a series of vascular hypoechoic nodules (*arrows*). Ultrasound-guided biopsy proved recurrent disease. Lesions were stable for more than 1 year at follow-up as patient declined surgery, having had thyroidectomy and two prior lymph node dissections.

cases of positive diagnostic findings and the surgical approach is dictated by the ultrasound findings.[53–55] As is the case with all ultrasound examinations, scans are operator dependent, and this procedure does have a learning curve.

We believe that ultrasound is a better technique than either CT or MRI and represents the most optimal method of postoperative surveillance in experienced hands. Lymph nodes in the neck are beautifully depicted by ultrasound and should be sought in the jugular chains and the thyroid bed bilaterally. Sonography is sufficiently sensitive that positive nodes occasionally may be encountered in patients who are thyroglobulin negative.[56,57] Exact location of identified adenopathy should be conveyed to the surgeon and

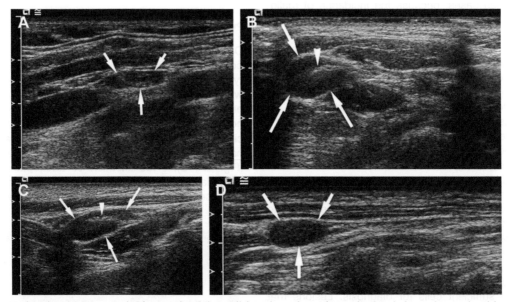

Fig. 12. (*A–D*) Benign cervical adenopathy. (*A*) Small lymph node with a cylindrical shape (*arrows*). Although a clearly defined echogenic fatty hilar region is not identified, small nodes with an elongate shape are common and can be assumed to be benign. Transverse (*B*) and longitudinal (*C*) sections through a relatively large cervical node (*arrows*) are shown in a patient with a history of thyroidectomy for papillary carcinoma. Note that the node is longer than it is wide and contains the presence of an echogenic fatty hilar region (*arrowheads*). (*D*) Indeterminate lymph node in a different patient with a history of thyroidectomy and papillary carcinoma but no prior imaging. Image shows a cervical lymph node that is likely benign based on shape but is somewhat rounder than the node shown in (*A*). It also does not have an echogenic hilus. Follow-up should be considered in such nodes that are likely benign but less confidently so than the node shown in (*A*).

specifically outlined in the report. We rely on the anatomic classification noted by Som and colleagues[58] in describing the level of the potentially abnormal lymph nodes (see **Fig. 1**). The recent article by Sheth and Hamper[15] also offers an excellent guide to nodal levels that is well adapted to the ultrasound examination.

For the most part, nodal anatomy is divided into the central compartment (nodal levels I, II, and VI) and lateral compartments (nodal levels II, III, and IV and the more lateral level V). The central compartment contains the thyroid bed and the paratracheal and paraesophageal lymph nodes and essentially comprises the area between the trachea and common carotid arteries. This area is normally "empty" in postthyroidectomy patients (**Fig. 10**), and any tissue identified in this area should be considered a recurrence until proven otherwise and biopsy performed (**Fig. 11A, B**). Level IA (submental) and level IB (submandibular) nodes are also included in the central

compartment but are rarely involved by metastatic thyroid cancers. The submandibular area, however, almost invariably contains benign nodes that may be fairly large, but because they are seldom involved by thyroid cancer they are only biopsied in unusual cases. The lateral cervical compartment contains superior, middle, and inferior jugular lymph nodes (levels II, III, and IV, respectively) and the dorsal cervical and supraclavicular nodes (levels VA and B).

The central and lateral compartments are divided by the common carotid sheath, which is the essential anatomic landmark for all sonographic cervical node examinations. The levels corresponding to the jugular venous chain (levels II–IV) are separated from level V nodes at the lateral border of the sternocleidomastoid muscle. Most metastatic lesions involve the thyroid bed or the mid or lower jugular venous lymph node chain (levels III and IV). Metastatic disease lateral to the sternocleidomastoid (level V) is relatively

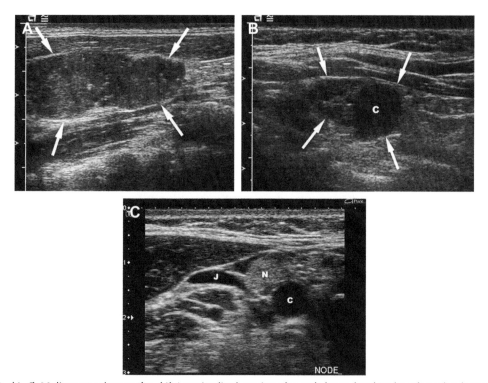

Fig. 13. (*A–C*) Malignant adenopathy. (*A*) Longitudinal section through large level VI lymph nodes (*arrows*) in a patient with a highly suspicious thyroid mass. Nodes are longer than they are wide but have an inhomogeneous internal echopattern and, most importantly, contain punctate echogenic foci typical of psammomatous calcifications of metastatic papillary carcinoma. Patient underwent thyroidectomy and lymph node dissection. (*B*) Level III node in patient with thyroidectomy for papillary carcinoma. Note cystic area in inferior portion of node (C), another finding that is highly suspicious for recurrent papillary carcinoma. Although biopsy should be directed toward solid portion of lymph node, sensitivity has been shown to improve in such cases with addition of evaluation for the presence of thyroglobulins. (*C*) Level III node in patient with thyroidectomy for papillary carcinoma. Note relatively homogeneous high level echogenicity of this node (N), which lies between the common carotid artery (C) and jugular vein (J). Ultrasound-guided biopsy results were positive for papillary carcinoma.

unusual. Recurrent disease in patients with differentiated thyroid carcinomas almost invariably is found ipsilateral to the original lesion. Patients with medullary thyroid carcinoma may present with contralateral or mediastinal disease.[59] Most authorities would recommend follow-up imaging at 6 and 12 months and yearly thereafter for 5 years.[26,60]

Although sensitive to the presence of adenopathy, imaging techniques are not specific, and differentiation between benign and malignant nodes may be difficult. For the most part, lymph nodes with an echogenic center are typically benign, as are oval or cylindrical nodes. Adenopathy at or above the level of the bifurcation (level II) and extending into the submandibular region (level IB) is also usually benign (**Fig. 12**A–C). Signs of malignant adenopathy include the presence of internal calcifications (an almost certain sign of recurrent papillary carcinoma), cystic or partially cystic nodes, and echogenic nodes (**Fig. 13**A, B).[15,61–63] Careful attention to technique is necessary to define internal calcifications that may be subtle and easily missed. Suspicion of malignancy also increases in lymph nodes with a more rounded appearance. Three-dimensional measurements of all lymph nodes are essential, and follow-up is often the key to metastatic involvement, with nodes that enlarge over time suggesting metastatic disease.

Shape may be quantified using a short to long axis ratio in which a measurement greater than or equal to 0.5 suggests that a node is involved with metastatic disease.[64] Essentially, the rounder the node, the greater the risk of involvement. Absolute size may be misleading, and the 1-cm cut-off applied to lymph nodes in the chest or abdomen cannot be applied to nodes in the neck. Even small nodes may harbor metastatic disease. The use of color in differentiating between benign and malignant adenopathy remains controversial. In a study by Steinkamp and colleagues,[65] 92% of reactive lymph nodes had significant hilar vascularity, and 84% of all metastatic nodes had peripheral vascularity. Approximately 79% of all lymphomatous nodes had mixed vascularity. We have not found the presence or absence of color to be of particular value in the differentiation between benign and malignant adenopathy in patients who have undergone thyroidectomy for cancer.

Biopsy of any suspicious lymph nodes is typically undertaken and the technique is similar to what was described previously for thyroid nodules (**Fig. 14**). The decision to perform biopsy in indeterminate nodes is often tempered by their size and number and the presence or absence of elevated

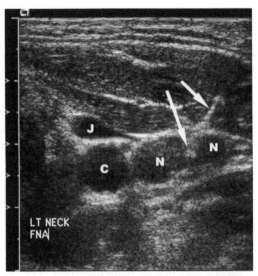

Fig. 14. Ultrasound-guided cervical node biopsy in patient with history of papillary carcinoma and prior thyroidectomy. Two hypoechoic nodes (N) are identified lateral to the left common carotid artery (C) and jugular vein (J). The needle (*arrows*) can be identified traversing the stenocleidomastoid muscle with tip in the nodes. Cytologic evaluation and thyroglobulin washing results were positive for papillary carcinoma.

thyroglobulin levels. Because differentiated thyroid carcinoma is a relatively indolent disease, indeterminate nodes simply may be followed over time. We have had patients with biopsy-proven nodal disease whose nodes have remained stable over several years. Lymph node biopsy may be more challenging than biopsy of thyroid nodules because the lymph nodes are often small and may be located adjacent to or even behind the carotid artery or jugular vein. It may be necessary to turn the patient's head toward or away from the transducer or even place the patient in a decubitus position in an attempt to gain access and avoid the adjacent vessels. Because thyroglobulin is only produced by thyroid tissue, either benign or malignant, its presence within an aspiration specimen of a lymph node essentially provides a positive diagnosis for metastasis and occasionally may be more sensitive than cytology alone.[66–68] Although we have had excellent results using cytology alone, we recently added a thyroglobulin evaluation to our nodal biopsy routine and believe that it is particularly important in patients with cystic adenopathy, in which cells may be difficult to obtain. This technique does not require an additional pass because the slides or washings themselves can be evaluated in the laboratory.

Percutaneous ethanol ablation of metastatic cervical lymph nodes in papillary thyroid carcinoma is gaining popularity. Many patients have undergone one—if not more—surgical procedure, including the initial thyroidectomy and subsequent lymph node dissections. These procedures render additional surgery difficult and may be further complicated by prior radioiodide or external radiation therapy. In such situations, repeat surgery is something that patients and their surgeons prefer to avoid. Because papillary carcinoma is a relatively indolent cancer, immediate treatment with complete removal of the node is not essential, and successful ablative treatment is monitored over time. For these reasons, percutaneous ablation represents an attractive alternative to repeat surgery.

In keeping with the technique described by Lewis and colleagues,[16] a 25-gauge needle is attached to a syringe containing approximately 1 mL of 95% ethanol. The area to be punctured is sterilized and instilled with local anesthesia. As opposed to routine biopsy in which subcutaneous anesthesia is sufficient, patients tend to experience less pain if local anesthesia is injected into the soft tissues surrounding lymph nodes to be ablated and not just into the skin. The needle is typically advanced to the deepest portion of the node, where a tiny amount (0.05–0 .1 mL) of ethanol is injected. One immediately sees a small echogenic area appear at the tip of the needle secondary to microbubbles in the injected alcohol. The needle can be repositioned and more injections performed until the physician believes the entire node has been treated. The procedure is terminated when the whole node has become echogenic (**Fig. 15**A–C). Larger nodes often require more than one session.

Patients can be brought back the following day and the injections repeated. Small injections are

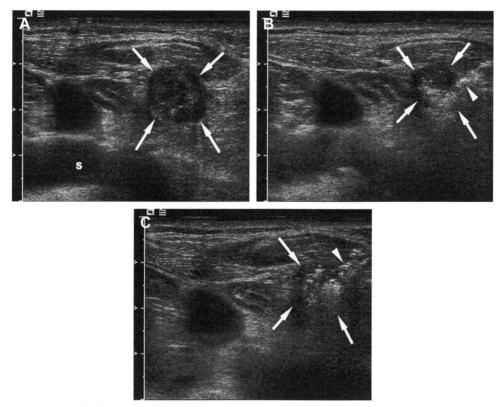

Fig. 15. (*A–C*) Ethanol ablation of metastatic lymph node in a 62-year-old man with history of thyroidectomy, multiple lymph node dissections, and local irradiation for recurrent papillary carcinoma. (*A*) Surveillance ultrasound revealed a single 1.5-cm right level IV node with internal calcifications (*arrows*) (SC, subclavian artery). Ultrasound-guided biopsy confirmed recurrent carcinoma. (*B*) Needle shaft (*arrowhead*) can be seen entering posterior portion of the node (*arrows*). Note that the posterior portion of the node is echogenic secondary to several injections of ethanol in this region. (*C*) Lymph node (*arrows*) is almost entirely obscured by high level echogenicity, suggesting that it has been injected throughout (*arrowhead* indicates needle shaft). Given the relatively large size of the node, the patient underwent a second similar procedure. Follow-up after 3 months demonstrated decrease in size of the node.

preferable to avoid extravasation beyond the limits of the lymph nodes, which may cause patients transient but significant pain. Unlike typical lymph nodes located in the jugular venous chain, percutaneous recurrence in the surgical beds is best avoided because of the increased potential for extravasation, pain, and potential recurrent laryngeal nerve transient paralysis (William Charboneau, MD, personal communication, 2008). Patients are typically followed at 3- and 6-month intervals after treatment, and repeat ablation procedures can be performed at that time if necessary. Success is suggested by decreasing size of the lymph node and absent perfusion by color Doppler. Thyroglobulin levels also should decrease with successful ablation. Newly found lymph nodes on subsequent follow ultrasound can be treated percutaneously. Recurrence of disease in successfully treated nodes seems to be uncommon.

SUMMARY

Ultrasound plays a pivotal role in the diagnosis and treatment of thyroid neoplasms. Although ultrasound evaluation of the thyroid and ultrasound-guided biopsy of thyroid nodules are commonplace, ultrasound monitoring and guided biopsy in postthyroidectomy patients have numerous advantages over competing techniques and are gaining in popularity. The nature of papillary cancer, with its propensity to spread slowly and locally, allows for ultrasound-guided ablation of limited recurrent nodal disease. This procedure can be performed safely and easily by radiologists and is gratifying because it can avoid repeated and difficult surgical procedures, and it should be advocated in selected patients.

REFERENCES

1. Tunbridge WMG, Evered DC, Hall R, et al. The spectrum of thyroid disease in a community: the Wickham survey. Clin Endocrinol 1977;7:481–93.
2. Vander JB, Gaston EA, Dawber TR. The significance of nontoxic thyroid nodules: final report of a 15-year study of the incidence of thyroid malignancy. Ann Intern Med 1968;69:537–40.
3. Jung HJ, Lim DJ, Baek KH, et al. Diagnostic value of ultrasonography to distinguish between benign and malignant lesions in the management of thyroid nodules. Thyroid 2007;18(5):461–6.
4. Ko HM, Jhu IK, Yang SH, et al. Clinicopathologic analysis of fine needle aspiration cytology of the thyroid: a review of 1,613 cases and correlation with histopathologic diagnoses. Acta Cytol 2003; 47:727–32.
5. Ravetto C, Colombo L, Dottorini ME. Usefulness of fine needle aspiration in the diagnosis of thyroid carcinoma: a retrospective study in 37,895 patients. Cancer 2000;90:357–63.
6. Amrikachi M, Ramzy I, Rubenfeld S, et al. Accuracy of fine-needle aspiration of thyroid. Arch Pathol Lab Med 2001;125:484–8.
7. Friedman M, Pacella BL. Total versus subtotal thyroidectomy: arguments, approaches and recommendations. Otolaryngol Clin North Am 1990;23: 413–27.
8. Hundahl SA, Fleming ID, Fremgen AM, et al. A national cancer data base report on 53,856 cases of thyroid carcinoma treated in the US, 1985–1995. Cancer 1998;83:2638–48.
9. Brierly JD, Panzarrella T, Tsang RW, et al. A comparison of different staging systems predictability of patient outcome: thyroid carcinoma as an example. Cancer 1997;79:2414–23.
10. Loevner LA, Kaplan SL, Cunnane ME, et al. Cross-sectional imaging of the thyroid gland. Neuroimaging Clin N Am 2008;18(3):445–61.
11. van den Brekel MW. Lymph node metastases: CT and MRI. Eur J Radiol 2000;33(3):230–8.
12. Pacini F, Molinaro E, Castagna MG, et al. Recombinant thyrotropin stimulated serum thyroglobulin combined with neck ultrasonography has the highest sensitivity in monitoring differentiated thyroid carcinoma. J Clin Endocrinol Metab 1999;84: 4549–53.
13. Baatenburg de Jong RJ, Rongen RJ, Verwoerd CD, et al. Ultrasound-guided fine-needle aspiration biopsy of neck nodes. Arch Otolaryngol Head Neck Surg 1991;117:402–4.
14. Sutton RT, Reading CC, Charboneau JW, et al. US guided biopsy of neck masses in postoperative management of patients with thyroid cancer. Radiology 1988;168:769–72.
15. Sheth S, Hamper UM. Role of sonography after total thyroidectomy for thyroid cancer. Ultrasound Q 2008;24:147–54.
16. Lewis BD, Hay ID, Charboneau JW, et al. Percutaneous ethanol injection for treatment of cervical lymph node metastasis in patients with thyroid carcinoma. AJR Am J Roentgenol 2002;178:699–704.
17. Johnson NA, Tublin ME. Post operative surveillance of differentiated thyroid carcinoma: rationale, techniques and controversies. Radiology 2008;249: 429–44.
18. Sherman SI. Thyroid carcinoma. Lancet 2003;361: 501–11.
19. Tyler DS, Winchester DJ, Caraway NP, et al. Towards improving the utility of fine needle aspiration biopsy for the diagnosis of thyroid tumors. Surgery 1994; 116:1054–60.
20. Tan GH, Gharib H. Thyroid incidentalomas: management approaches to non-palpable nodules

discovered incidentally on thyroid imaging. Ann Intern Med 1997;126:226–31.

21. Mandel SJ. A 64 year old woman with a thyroid nodule. JAMA 2004;292:2632–42.

22. Hegedus L. Clinical practice: the thyroid nodule. N Engl J Med 2004;351:1764–71.

23. Jemal A, Murray T, Ward E, et al. Cancer statistics 2005. CA Cancer J Clin 2005;55:10–30.

24. Hodgson NC, Button J, Solorzano CC. Thyroid cancer: is the incidence still increasing? Ann Surg Oncol 2004;11:1093–7.

25. American Association of Clinical Endocrinologists/ Associazione Medici Endocarinologi Task Force on Thyroid Nodules. Medical guidelines for clinical practice for the diagnosis and management of thyroid nodules. Endocr Pract 2006;12:65–102.

26. Cooper DS, Doherty GM, Haugen RT, et al. Management guidelines for patients with thyroid nodules and differentiated thyroid cancer. Thyroid 2006;16:109–41.

27. Frates MC, Benson CB, Charboneau JW, et al. Management of thyroid nodules discovered at US Society of Radiologists in Ultrasound consensus statement. Radiology 2005;237:794–800.

28. Hermus AR. Clinical manifestations and treatment of nontoxic diffuse and nodular goiter. In: Braverman LE, Utiger RD, Ingbar SH, et al, editors. Werner and Ingbar's the hyroid: a fundamental and clinical text. Philadelphia: Lippincott Williams & Wilkins; 2000. p. 867.

29. Hegedus L, Bonnema SJ, Bennedbaek FN. Management of simple nodular goiter: current status and future perspectives. Endocr Rev 2003;24:102–32.

30. Marqusee E, Benson CB, Frates MC, et al. Usefulness of ultrasonography in the management of nodular thyroid disease. Ann Intern Med 2000;1339:696–700.

31. Papini E, Guglielmi R, Bianchini A, et al. Risk of malignancy in non-palpable thyroid nodules: predictive value of ultrasound and color Doppler features. J Clin Endocrinol Metab 2002;87:1941–6.

32. Katz JF, Kane RA, Reyes J, et al. Thyroid nodules: sonographic–pathologic correlation. Radiology 1984;151:741–5.

33. Brkljacic B, Cuk V, Tomic-Brzac H, et al. Ultrasonic evaluation of benign and malignant nodules in echographically multinodular thyroids. J Clin Ultrasound 1994;22:71–6.

34. Reading CC, Charboneau JW, Hays ID, et al. Sonography of thyroid nodules: a "classic pattern" diagnostic approach. Ultrasound Q 2005;21:157–65.

35. Kim EK, Park CS, Chung WY, et al. New sonographic criteria for recommending fine-needle aspiration biopsy of nonpalpable solid nodules of the thyroid. AJR Am J Roentgenol 2002;178:687–91.

36. Park CH, Rothermel FJ, Judge DM. Unusual calcification in mixed papillary and follicular carcinoma of the thyroid gland. Radiology 1976;119:554–8.

37. Kim MJ, Kim EK, Kwak JY, et al. Differentiation of thyroid nodules with macrocalcifications: role of suspicious sonographic findings. J Ultrasound Med 2008;27:1179–84.

38. Wang N, Xu Y, Ge C, et al. Association of sonographically detected calcification with thyroid carcinoma. Head Neck 2006;28:1077–83.

39. Kim BM, Kim MJ, Kim EK. Sonographic differentiation of thyroid nodules with eggshell calcifications. J Ultrasound Med 2008;27:1425–30.

40. Ahuja A, Chick W, King W, et al. Clinical significance of the comet-tail artifact in thyroid ultrasound. J Clin Ultrasound 1996;24:129–33.

41. Stavros AT, Thickman D, Rapp CL, et al. Solid breast nodules: use of sonography to distinguish between benign and malignant lesions. Radiology 1995;196:123–34.

42. Propper RA, Skolnick ML, Weinstein BJ, et al. The nonspecificity of the thyroid halo sign. J Clin Ultrasound 1980;8:129–32.

43. Holden A. The role of colour and duplex Doppler ultrasound in the assessment of thyroid nodules. Australas Radiol 1995;39:343–9.

44. Shimamoto K, Endo T, Ishigaki T, et al. Thyroid nodules: evaluation with color Doppler ultrasonography. J Ultrasound Med 1993;12:673–8.

45. Pacini F, Elisei R, Capezzone M, et al. Contralateral papillary thyroid cancer is frequent at completion thyroidectomy with no difference in low and high risk patients. Thyroid 2001;11:877–81.

46. Ylagan LR, Farkas T, Dehner LP. Fine needle aspiration biopsy of the thyroid: a cytohistologic correlation and study of discrepant cases. Thyroid 2004;14:35–41.

47. Baloch ZW, Fleisher S, Li Volsi VA, et al. Diagnosis of "follicular neoplasm": a gray zone in thyroid fine needle aspiration cytology. Diagn Cytopathol 2002;26:41–4.

48. Erdem E, Gulcelik MA, Kuru B, et al. Comparison of completion thyroidectomy and primary surgery for differentiated thyroid carcinoma. Eur J Surg Oncol 2003;29:747–9.

49. Fraker DL. Thyroid tumors. In: DeVita V Jr, Hellman S, Rosenberg S, editors. Cancer: principles and practice of oncology. Philadelphia: Lippincott-Raven; 1997. p. 1629–52.

50. Chow LS, Gharib H, Goellner JR, et al. Nondiagnostic thyroid fine-needle aspiration cytology: management dilemmas. Thyroid 2001;11:1147–51.

51. McHenry CR, Walfish PG, Rosen IB. Nondiagnostic fine needle aspiration biopsy: a dilemma in management of nodular thyroid disease. Am Surg 1993;59:415–9.

52. Khoo TK, Baker CH, Hallinger-Johnson J, et al. Comparison of ultrasound-guided fine-needle aspiration biopsy with core-needle biopsy in the evaluation of thyroid nodules. Endocr Pract 2008;14(4):426–31.

53. Kouvaraki MA, Shapiro SE, Fornage BD, et al. Role of preoperative ultrasonography in the surgical management of patients with thyroid cancer. Surgery 2003;134:946–54.

54. Gemsenjager E, Perren A, Seifert B, et al. Lymph node surgery in papillary thyroid carcinoma. J Am Coll Surg 2003;197:182–90.

55. Ito Y, Tomoda C, Uruno T, et al. Preoperative ultrasonographic examination for lymph node metastasis: usefulness when designing lymph node dissection for papillary microcarcinoma. World J Surg 2004; 28(5):498–501.

56. Torlontano M, Attard M, Crocetti U, et al. Follow-up of low risk patients with papillary thyroid cancer: role of neck ultrasonography in detecting lymph node metastases. J Clin Endocrinol Metab 2004;89(7): 3402–7.

57. Shin JH, Han BK, Ko EY, et al. Sonographic findings in the surgical bed after thyroidectomy: comparison of recurrent tumors and nonrecurrent lesions. J Ultrasound Med 2007;26(10):1359–66.

58. Som PM, Curtin HD, Mancuso AA. Imaging-based nodal classification for evaluation of neck metastatic adenopathy. Am J Roentgenol 2000;174(3):837–44.

59. Machens A, Hinze R, Thomusch O, et al. Pattern of nodal metastasis for primary and reoperative thyroid cancer. World J Surg 2002;26(1):22–8.

60. Pacini F, Schlumberger M, Dralle H, et al. European consensus for the management of patients with differentiated thyroid carcinoma of the follicular epithelium. Eur J Endocrinol 2006;154(6): 787–803.

61. Chan JM, Shin LK, Jeffrey LB. Ultrasonography of abnormal neck lymph nodes. Ultrasound Q 2007; 23:47–54.

62. Ahuja AT, Ying M, Yang WT, et al. The use of sonography in differentiating cervical lymphomatous lymph nodes from cervical metastatic lymph nodes. Clin Radiol 1996;51:186–90.

63. Sakai F, Kiyono K, Sone S, et al. Ultrasonic evaluation of cervical metastatic lymphadenopathy. J Ultrasound Med 1988;7:305–10.

64. Van den Brekel MWM, Castelijns JA, Snow GB. The size of lymph nodes in the neck on sonograms as a radiologic criterion for metastasis: how reliable is it? AJNR Am J Neuroradiol 1998;19:695–700.

65. Steinkamp HJ, Muesselmann M, Bock JC, et al. Differential diagnosis of lymph node lesions: a semi-quantitative approach with colour Doppler ultrasound. Br J Radiol 1998;71:828–33.

66. Cunha N, Rodrigues F, Curado F, et al. Thyroglobulin detection in fine-needle aspirates of cervical lymph nodes: a technique for the diagnosis of metastatic differentiated thyroid cancer. Eur J Endocrinol 2007;157(1):101–7.

67. Baskin HJ. Detection of recurrent papillary thyroid carcinoma by thyroglobulin assessment in the needle washout after fine-needle aspiration of suspicious lymph nodes. Thyroid 2004;14(11):959–63.

68. Cignarelli M, Ambrosi A, Marino A, et al. Diagnostic utility of thyroglobulin detection in fine-needle aspiration of cervical cystic metastatic lymph nodes from papillary thyroid cancer with negative cytology. Thyroid 2003;13(12):1163–7.

Ultrasound-guided Biopsies of Peripleural Lung Lesions

Shannon M. Gulla, MD, Hisham Tchelepi, MD,
Brent T. Steadman, MD, PhD, Hollins P. Clark, MD*

KEYWORDS

- Image fusion • Lung biopsy • Peripheral lung biopsy
- Sonographic guidance • Ultrasound-guided

Ultrasound-guided biopsies of lesions in solid tissues of the neck, abdomen, pelvis, and subcutaneous soft tissues are now common. Intrathoracic biopsies typically are reserved for CT guidance given the inability of ultrasound to image through air. Peripheral lung lesions in contact with the pleural surface are visible by ultrasound, however, and so are candidates for ultrasound-guided biopsy. Success rates for sonographic-guided sampling of mediastinal lesions are as high as 71% to 100%, whereas rates for peripheral lung lesions are even more convincing at 89% to 98% when using core biopsies.[1] This article reviews the advantages and disadvantages of ultrasound-guided biopsy for peripleural lung lesions, describes appropriate technique, and briefly discusses management of complications.

ADVANTAGES OF ULTRASOUND-GUIDED PERIPHERAL LUNG BIOPSY

Despite the nearly universal availability of sonographic equipment, CT guidance is nearly always chosen for lung and mediastinal biopsies. Using sonographic guidance frees the CT scanner for diagnostic use, or for procedures in which it is specifically required.

Because sonographic equipment is relatively mobile, ultrasound-guided biopsies can be performed in the patient's room, particularly in situations where infection control might be a concern. This advantage is helpful for diagnostic and therapeutic thoracentesis and drainage catheter placement (**Fig. 1**), and can be adapted for peripleural tissue diagnosis.

With a significant overall increase in the use of imaging in patient care, awareness regarding patient radiation dose is necessary. Every effort must be made to choose the appropriate study and perform the examination with the least radiation possible to solve the clinical problem. The use of ultrasound for biopsies instead of CT or fluoroscopy decreases both the patient and the physician's cumulative radiation dose. Repeated imaging can be obtained throughout the procedure without concern for dose to radiosensitive tissues.

Because sonographic guidance is "real-time," the biopsy needle tip can be visualized throughout the procedure. This improves safety, particularly when patients cannot follow directions or suspend respiration for accurate needle placement as is necessary with tomographic guidance (**Fig. 2**). Because the target lesion and needle remain in the imaging plane despite respiratory variability, this attribute is particularly useful with smaller lesions that change positions during the respiratory cycle. CT fluoroscopy, not yet widely available, likewise compensates for respiratory variation, although at the cost of using ionizing radiation.

With traditional methods for biopsy guidance, patients are generally supine, prone, or decubitus. With sonographic guidance there is greater flexibility. For example, if a patient has difficulty remaining prone for an extended period of time,

Department of Radiology, Wake Forest University School of Medicine, Medical Center Boulevard, Winston-Salem, NC 27157, USA
* Corresponding author.
E-mail address: hclarck@wfubmc.edu (H.P. Clark).

Ultrasound Clin 4 (2009) 17–24
doi:10.1016/j.cult.2009.03.005
1556-858X/09/$ – see front matter © 2009 Published by Elsevier Inc.

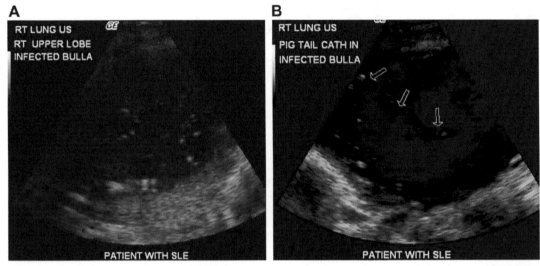

Fig. 1. Sonographic evaluation of infected right apical bulla (*A*) with subsequent placement of drainage catheter (*B*).

the procedure can be performed with the patient leaning forward over a support. Similarly, procedures can be performed with the patient upright and supported. This is particularly helpful in patients with orthopnea. Ultrasound's flexibility also permits rapid and uncomplicated change in patient positioning to facilitate sampling of multiple lesions (**Fig. 3**). If, for example, biopsy of a selected lesion does not provide diagnostic results, the patient can be repositioned as needed to sample an alternative site.

Detection of chest wall invasion can be critical for cancer staging and for selection of an optimal biopsy site. In particular, lung lesions that extend into the peripheral tissues of the chest are more likely to be fixed, decreasing the risk for

pneumothorax associated with biopsy. Ultrasound is well-suited to determining chest wall invasion. Bandi and colleagues[2] compared ultrasound with CT in 90 patients with surgical correlation, and reported better sensitivity (89% for ultrasound, 42% for CT) with excellent specificity (95% for ultrasound, 100% for CT) in detecting chest wall invasion (**Fig. 4**).

DISADVANTAGES OF ULTRASOUND-GUIDED PERIPHERAL LUNG BIOPSY

Although sonographic equipment is widely available, it is less frequently used for thoracic interventions. The exception to this is thoracentesis, for which sonographic imaging is routinely used

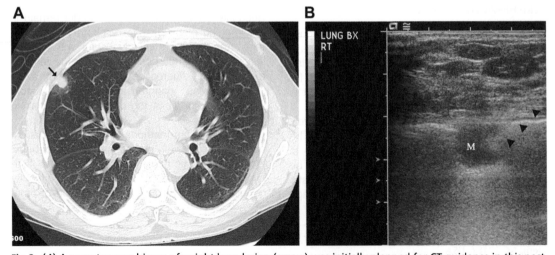

Fig. 2. (*A*) A percutaneous biopsy of a right lung lesion (*arrow*) was initially planned for CT guidance in this post-transplant patient. (*B*) Needle tract (*arrowheads*) from sonographic biopsy, ultimately performed because of variability in position of the hypoechoic mass (M). Final pathologic diagnosis was *Cryptococcus* and the patient was managed with appropriate medical therapy.

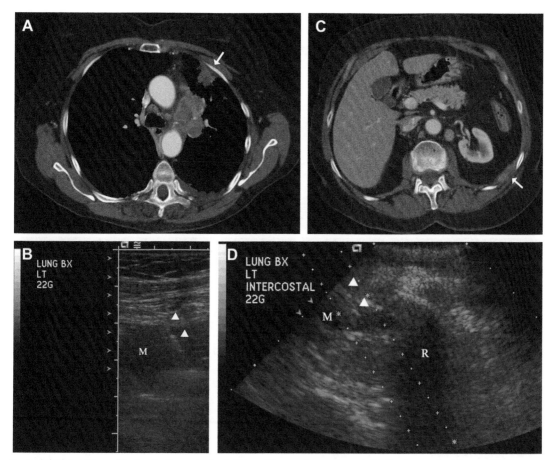

Fig. 3. (A) Pleural-based lesion in the anterior left hemithorax (*arrow*) was initially chosen for biopsy. (B) The mass (M) and needle tract (*arrowheads*) were clearly demonstrated during fine-needle aspiration. (C) Because of insufficient cellularity, a separate posterior intercostal lesion (*arrow*) was sampled. (D) The hypoechoic mass (M) can be seen on the lateral aspect of the image, with needle tract (*arrowheads*) closely following the sonographic needle guide. Adjacent rib shadowing (R) was avoided. Final pathologic diagnosis was adenocarcinoma.

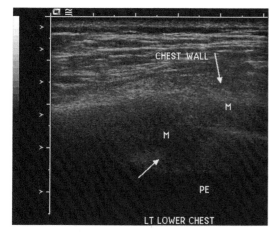

Fig. 4. Periphery (*arrows*) of the mass (M) can be readily identified extending into the soft tissues of the chest wall in this patient with a malignant pleural effusion (PE).

both preprocedurally for marking, or intraprocedurally for monitoring needle course. Interventionalists traditionally have been more comfortable with CT guidance for biopsies, particularly in the thorax. Ultrasound-directed biopsies require facility with real-time imaging of needle placement, which necessitates dedicated training, experience, and hand-eye coordination.

Before scheduling a biopsy under sonographic guidance, CT has usually been performed for diagnosis or staging. The CT helps to determine the most accessible lesion for the safest biopsy. Ultrasound-guided lung and chest wall biopsies are typically reserved for those lesions with a pre-biopsy high probability of neoplastic disease (**Fig. 5**). If there is reason to suspect that the lesion could be infectious or inflammatory, and might have improved in the interval between diagnosis and biopsy, a repeat CT may be necessary to assess change (**Fig. 6**). Although the lesion can

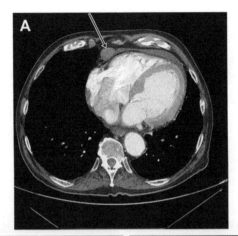

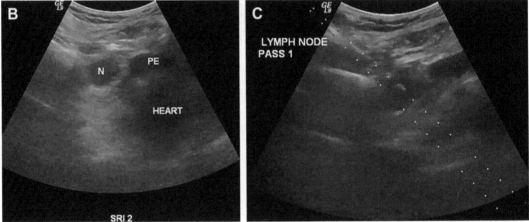

Fig. 5. Pericardial lymph node (*arrow*) seen on CT (*A*) in a patient with colon cancer was evaluated with ultrasound (*B*) for subsequent sonographic biopsy (*C*). As seen on CT, the target node (N) was immediately adjacent to pericardial effusion (PE) on sonographic evaluation. Pathologic diagnosis was consistent with metastatic disease.

be measured sonographically and compared with measurements from the CT examination, comparison using the same modality is preferred.

To create an image, ultrasound requires a medium through which an acoustic beam can be transmitted, reflected, and recorded. Unfortunately, aerated lung is not such a medium. Consequently, many lung lesions are not accessible for ultrasound-guided biopsy. Lesions surrounded by aerated lung or protected by overlying osseous structures cannot be sampled.

Because smaller nodules are more difficult to visualize under ultrasound, early studies with sonographic guidance excluded lesions less than 3 cm in size.[3] More recently, however, investigators targeting lesions less than 3 cm in size[4] demonstrated this technique could be accurate, safe, and effective.

Ultrasound-guided procedures, including lung biopsies, have the same complication rate as those performed with CT imaging guidance, as

low as 5%.[1] Pneumothorax can be more difficult to manage, however, under ultrasound. A large pneumothorax could completely obscure the biopsy site such that premature termination of the procedure may be necessary. In this situation, the procedure could require conversion to CT guidance for chest tube placement or biopsy completion.

ULTRASOUND-GUIDED PERIPHERAL LUNG BIOPSY TECHNIQUE

An appropriate patient for ultrasound-guided lung biopsy has a soft tissue mass involving or abutting the pleural surface. Nodules entirely surrounded by aerated lung cannot be biopsied sonographically. Small lesions less than 3 cm in size can be successfully biopsied, but larger lesions with greater chest wall involvement are the ideal candidates.

Before scheduling the procedure, a review of the patient's medical record and relevant imaging

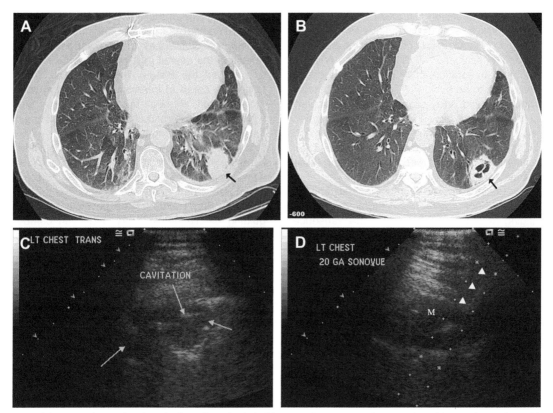

Fig. 6. (A) CT performed 9 days before the scheduled biopsy demonstrated a peripheral lesion (arrow) readily accessible for sonographic percutaneous biopsy. (B) Repeat CT acquired on the day of the biopsy demonstrated interval cavitation (arrow). (C) Hyperechoic areas of cavitation (arrows) were clearly visible sonographically. (D) Needle tract (arrowheads) from multiple fine-needle aspirates of the mass (M) are clearly visualized. The final diagnosis was adenocarcinoma.

should be performed. Medical review should include evaluation of the patient's laboratory studies. Coagulation ratios, hematocrits, and platelet counts should be evaluated and corrected as needed. Review of the patient's record should also include a review of previous imaging in general and CT in particular. This review can confirm the necessity of the procedure and the appropriateness of the guiding modality. In some instances, a biopsy previously scheduled for tomographic guidance can be scheduled instead with sonographic guidance. A previous CT is important, however, for localization of the lesion most amenable to biopsy. Repeat imaging might also be warranted before sonographic biopsy because documented improvement of an infectious or inflammatory lesion obviates the procedure (see **Fig. 6**).

Informed consent is an important part of the patient's preprocedural care and should detail the procedure in nonmedical terms to ensure adequate patient comprehension. The patient should also be made aware of alternatives to the procedure, if any. As in other interventional procedures, the consent process requires a discussion of the risks, which include bleeding, infection, damage to adjacent structures, pneumothorax, and the potential need for a chest tube or emergency surgery. The discussion should also mention the possibility of conversion to a CT-guided procedure in the event of a technical failure or complication.

Patient positioning can be variable for sonographic-guided biopsies. Prone or supine positioning offers the best patient stability to prevent discomfort and resultant patient movement. Some patients, however, require nonstandard positioning to perform the biopsy. If necessary, biopsies can be performed with the patient seated and the head of the bed elevated to support the patient's back. Alternatively, tissue samples can be acquired with the patient leaning over a table or other adequate support.

Once the patient is positioned, a sonographic survey of the target and surrounding tissues should be performed. Use of a higher megahertz probe improves lesion visualization because the target usually is relatively superficial. Preprocedural imaging with a linear or curvilinear probe allows appropriate evaluation of the lesion and adjacent structures. In addition, color Doppler can identify vasculature to be avoided (**Fig. 7**). Subsequently, a tightly curved array probe can be particularly useful because it allows a steeper needle trajectory, which is frequently necessary for smaller pleural-based lesions. Because of their size, linear or curvilinear probes allow only shallow angle needle trajectories.

The usual transverse and sagittal imaging planes are not common for thoracic biopsies. Imaging must be performed with the transducer parallel to the adjacent ribs. Overlying rib shadows can obscure the lesion and surrounding structures, including vasculature. If the transducer is not properly positioned with respect to the ribs (see **Fig. 3**D), the acoustic window is effectively decreased. Using an oblique intercostal orientation rather than the standard axial or sagittal affords optimal simultaneous depiction of the target lesion and the needle.

Initial adjustments of the time-gain compensation can be necessary to compensate for acoustic impedance differences among various tissues. Adjusting the overall gain might also be required to optimize the image. The focal zone should target the depth of interest. Multiple focal zones may be used, although this increases scan time, which may not be optimal during real-time imaging for percutaneous lung biopsy.

The biopsy can be performed with or without ultrasound needle guidance hardware and software, which maintain the needle trajectory at a predetermined angle (see **Figs. 3**D, **5**C, **6**D, and **7**C). Some experienced physicians find the guiding needle unnecessary and even cumbersome. The free-hand technique allows approach to the lesion from multiple angles relative to the transducer (see **Figs. 2**B and **3**B; **Fig. 8**). With either technique, the needle should be kept in the imaging plane throughout the procedure to be certain of the position and minimize damage to adjacent structures.

Samples can be obtained using either fine-needle aspiration or core biopsy, with or without

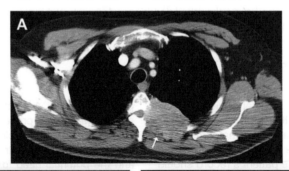

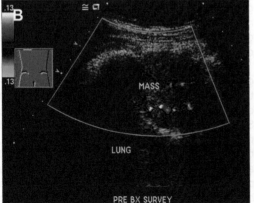

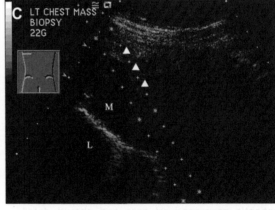

Fig. 7. (*A*) Biopsy of a large peripleural mass (*arrow*) was requested to document metastatic disease. (*B*) Prebiopsy sonographic imaging with color Doppler demonstrates increased vascularity of the tumor. (*C*) Biopsy tract (*arrowheads*) through the mass (M) was maintained in the periphery of the lesion to avoid vascularity and adjacent lung (L). The final pathologic diagnosis was renal cell carcinoma.

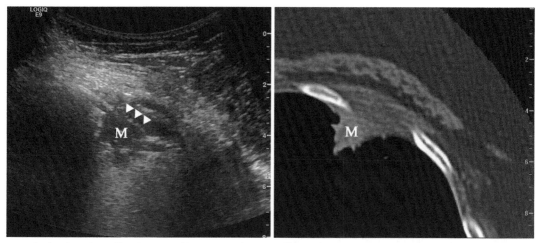

Fig. 8. Fusion imaging offers improved lesion visualization allowing real-time correlation between the ultrasound for biopsy (*left*) and screening CT scan (*right*). Needle tract (*arrowheads*) can be followed into the mass (M) with corresponding changes in fused CT.

a coaxial system. In institutions with cytopathology available for on-site consultation, fine-needle aspirates are often adequate for diagnosis. Core biopsies may be necessary, however, when special stains are needed or in the setting of lymphoma.[5]

Imaging is continuous throughout the biopsy under sonographic guidance. Although pneumothorax can be difficult to discern, the lack of sliding motion that is seen with normal aerated lung is a good diagnostic sign. "Comet tail" artifacts can also be seen in normally aerated lung, but are absent in a pneumothorax.[1]

Postbiopsy chest radiography should be performed routinely, even if no pneumothorax is suspected by ultrasound. If there is no evidence of pneumothorax or hemorrhage on serial radiographs, outpatients are released. They should be informed that blood-tinged sputum is common postbiopsy, but copious hemoptysis should not occur. Additionally, shortness of breath or chest pain should prompt a visit to the nearest emergency department.

MANAGEMENT OF IMMEDIATE POSTPROCEDURAL COMPLICATIONS

Pneumothorax has been reported in up to 61% of percutaneous CT-guided biopsies, causing chest pain, dyspnea, and decreased oxygen saturation.[6,7] Most postprocedural pneumothoraces develop within the first hour after the procedure and might not be visible immediately after the biopsy. Occasionally, this complication is delayed, occurring 24 hours after the biopsy.[6] Although small pneumothoraces can be monitored on an outpatient basis, large or worsening pneumothoraces often require a chest tube placed to wall suction, water seal, or a Heimlich valve, depending on the severity of the air leak. Chest tubes in this setting can usually be removed in 1 to 2 days, even in patients with emphysema.

A small amount of focal pulmonary hemorrhage is common in lung biopsies and is reported in 5% to 17% of biopsies, with hemoptysis reported in 1% to 5% of patients. On CT, pulmonary hemorrhage creates a zone of airspace opacity adjacent to the biopsy site, but the bleeding can be less obvious sonographically. Generally, pulmonary hemorrhage and hemoptysis are self-limited. More significant hemorrhage or hemoptysis can also occur, particularly if the lesion is more than 2 cm from the pleura.[6,8] Patients rarely require fluid resuscitation and oxygen.

Hemothorax is a rare complication from damage to adjacent vasculature, such as an intercostal or internal mammary artery.[9] Supportive care including fluids and oxygen can be helpful. Ultimately, significant bleeding resulting in hemothorax may require the assistance of interventional radiology and vascular or thoracic surgery.

Air embolism as a result of percutaneous lung biopsy is only rarely reported and so the exact incidence is unknown.[6,9,10] Reports of these cases include some fatalities.[6,7,11] Air embolism could result when a needle is placed into a small pulmonary vein and air is inadvertently aspirated on removal of the stylet. With supine and prone patient positioning, air is less likely to enter the cranial circulation as it moves into the least dependent location. Placing the patient in the left lateral decubitus position or Trendelenburg position can be necessary if a residual air collection remains in the left heart.

FUTURE OF SONOGRAPHIC PERIPLEURAL BIOPSIES

Recent technologic advances allow fusion of imaging modalities. Fusion of positron emission tomography with CT is now common. Fusion of ultrasound with CT is relatively new, however, and definitely not as widespread as positron emission tomography–CT. Images from a recent CT are uploaded into the ultrasound machine, after which the ultrasound images can be fused with the previous screening study (see **Fig. 8**). As the ultrasound probe is moved over the patient, the corresponding CT image adjusts in real-time. This new technology provides the spatial resolution and anatomic detail of CT with the real-time needle guidance provided by ultrasound. Furthermore, the fused sonographic biopsy is portable without the use of additional ionizing radiation.

SUMMARY

Ultrasound is an alternative to the traditional CT guidance most often used for lung biopsies. Although not appropriate for all thoracic biopsies, this technique can be a safe and effective choice for peripleural lung lesions. As emerging technologies, such as image fusion, gain wider acceptance, ultrasound-guided thoracic biopsy will be more than a footnote.

REFERENCES

1. Middleton WD, Teefey SA, Dahiya N. Ultrasound-guided chest biopsies. Ultrasound Q 2006;22(4): 241–52.
2. Bandi V, Lunn W, Ernst A, et al. Ultrasound vs. CT in detecting chest wall invasion by tumor. Chest 2008; 133(4):881–6.
3. Yang PC, Chang DB, Yu CJ, et al. Ultrasound-guided core biopsy of thoracic tumors. Am Rev Respir Dis 1992;146:763–7.
4. Liao WY, Chen MZ, Chang YL, et al. US-guided transthoracic cutting biopsy for peripheral thoracic lesions less than 3 cm in diameter. Radiology 2000;217:685–91.
5. Ahrar K, Wallace M, Javadi S, et al. Mediastinal, hilar, pleural image-guided biopsy: current practice and techniques. Semin Respir Crit Care Med 2008; 29:350–60.
6. Manhire A, Charig M, Clelland C, et al. Guidelines for radiologically guided lung biopsy. Thorax 2003; 58(11):920–36.
7. Kodama F, Ogawa T, Hashimoto M, et al. Fatal air embolism as a complication of CT-guided needle biopsy of the lung. J Comput Assist Tomogr 1999; 23(6):949–51.
8. Yeow KM, See LC, Lui KW, et al. Risk factors for pneumothorax and bleeding after CT-guided percutaneous coaxial cutting needle biopsy of lung lesions. J Vasc Interv Radiol 2001;12(11): 1305–12.
9. Glassberg RM, Sussman SK. Life-threatening hemorrhage due to percutaneous transthoracic intervention: importance of the internal mammary artery. AJR Am J Roentgenol 1990;154(1):47–9.
10. Klein JS, Salomon G, Stewart EA. Transthoracic needle biopsy with a coaxially placed 20-gauge automated cutting needle: results in 122 patients. Radiology 1996;198(3):715–20.
11. Tolly TL, Feldmeier JE, Czarnecki D. Air embolism complicating percutaneous lung biopsy. AJR Am J Roentgenol 1988;150(3):555–6.

Ultrasound and Abdominal Intervention: New Luster on an Old Gem

David D. Childs, MD*, Hisham Tchelepi, MD

KEYWORDS

- Ultrasound • Abdomen • Intervention • Biopsy
- Drainage • Fusion imaging

Sonographic guidance for abdominal intervention-al applications is certainly not a new concept, but it is an often forgotten tool. As pointed out by Dodd and coworkers,[1] many radiologists have tradition-ally been more familiar with computed tomog-raphy (CT) as a needle guidance method. This is unfortunate, because ultrasound holds a number of advantages over CT. By providing real-time visualization, sonography provides for faster nee-dle traversal and the ability to more safely control the needle trajectory, avoiding vital structures, such as vessels. Sheafor and colleagues,[2] for example, found that biopsies performed on a phantom were significantly faster with ultra-sound guidance as compared with helical CT. Documentation of needle placement inside a lesion is also provided, minimizing diagnostic uncer-tainty. Ultrasound has been shown to be cheaper than CT. Kliewer and colleagues[3] showed that liver biopsies using sonographic guidance were 1.89 times less expensive than liver biopsies performed with CT guidance. A lack of ionizing radiation is also an important advantage, because CT's potential role in cancer induction has been high-lighted recently.[4] Portability is a strength, allowing interventions to be performed on critically ill patients who cannot be transported safely to the radiology department. Newer technology, such as fusion imaging (discussed later), has actually narrowed the gap between ultrasound and CT, allowing one to take advantage of both simultaneously.

TECHNOLOGY

There are three basic types of ultrasound probes available for use in sonography. The vector trans-ducer has a small footprint and relatively deep penetration of the sound beam, allowing needle passage through relatively "tight" acoustic windows, such as an intercostal approach. The major disadvantages are a relatively small field of view, especially in the near-field, and relatively low spatial resolution. Needle guides are available for this class of probes, but the needle tip is often not visualized until it has passed into the deeper tissues. This can become problematic if the radiol-ogist wishes to avoid more superficial structures, such as vessels or bowel. Lately, this has been improved by the development of newer high-reso-lution phased-array transducers with virtual convex providing the operator better resolution and wider field of view. These transducers are also capable of penetrating into the deeper tissues, making them ideal for small deep lesions. A phased-array curved transducer has a large footprint that necessitates a relatively large acoustic window, such as a subcostal approach to a liver lesion. The major advantages include good spatial resolution and a relatively large field of view, especially beneficial for visualizing the near-field. Needle guides are available for this class of probe, but because of the shape of the probe this often increases the distance from the guide to the skin. This is usually of no

Department of Radiology/MRI Building, Wake Forest University School of Medicine, Wake Forest University Baptist Medical Center, Medical Center Boulevard, Winston-Salem, NC 27157, USA
* Corresponding author.
E-mail address: dchilds@wfubmc.edu (D.D. Childs).

Ultrasound Clin 4 (2009) 25–43
doi:10.1016/j.cult.2009.03.004

consequence, although one must be vigilant to align the needle with the anesthetized patch of skin. Linear high-resolution probes are best for superficial structures, because they provide excellent spatial resolution at the expense of decreased image depth. Guides have also been developed for these probes, facilitating quick needle passage.

Color Doppler is a valuable tool that is universally available. It is quite useful in planning needle trajectory, minimizing the risk of damage to interposed vascular structures. It is equally efficacious as a screening tool for procedure-related complications, such as active bleeding or arteriovenous fistula (AVF).

For percutaneous sampling, one essentially has two options: fine needle aspiration (FNA) and core biopsy. The choice of needle depends on the suspected pathology, available pathology resources, operator experience, and patient factors. For instance, if no cytology service is available to review samples, a core specimen is useful. In the setting of coagulopathy or a suspected hypervascular tumor, such as hepatocellular carcinoma or renal call carcinoma metastasis, simple FNA may be a more prudent choice. FNA may also be preferable in situations where there are vessels or bowel in close proximity to the target, or when traversal of bowel is required, such as in biopsy of the pancreas. There is evidence that core specimens yield a higher and more consistent positive

diagnostic rate than fine-needle aspirates for abdominal lesions in adults[5] and children.[6] Hugosson and colleagues[6] did, however, show that the diagnostic yield of FNA increased directly with operator experience.

The newest ultrasound technology (fusion imaging) allows the operator to use CT, MR imaging, and ultrasound image data simultaneously. This technology uses image fusion, in which a previously acquired CT or MR imaging volumetric data set is "fused" to the gray-scale ultrasound image. A receiver device monitors the movement and position of the ultrasound transducer, which itself emits an electromagnetic signal. As the ultrasound probe is manipulated, the operator sees a traditional gray-scale image and the "matching" CT or MR image reconstructed in the same plane as the transducer (**Fig. 1**). This is especially useful for the biopsy of lesions that are more easily seen on CT or MR imaging than on ultrasound.

LIVER

Both native and transplant livers are easily accessible by sonographic guidance. Possible approaches include intercostal, subcostal, and epigastric. From the subcostal or epigastric approach, one must use caution to avoid the colon and stomach, respectively. Primary concerns for the intercostal approach include vascular injury

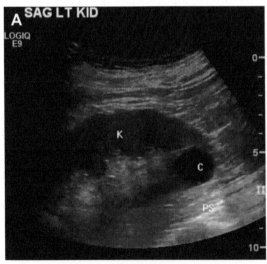 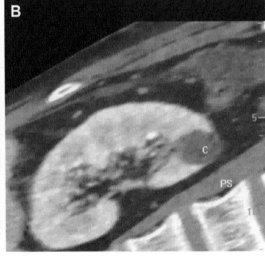

Fig. 1. Fused ultrasound-CT image (*A, B*) of a complex cyst in the lower pole of the right kidney. The image shows combined ultrasound and CT images as obtained on the ultrasound machine. The CT data have already been imported from the PACS system before ultrasound imaging. Using special software and hardware the CT images are fused with the ultrasound images during real-time scanning. The accuracy of such technique is within 3 mm and is dependent on precise selection of reference anatomic points on both the CT and ultrasound images. Refer to text for further details about fusion technology. C, cyst; K, kidney; PS, psoas muscle.

and pneumothorax. Staying below the twelfth rib posteriorly or the tenth rib laterally should avoid pleural transgression,[7] although a transpleural route usually does not result in pneumothorax if aerated lung is avoided. The needle should not scrape the inferior margin of the rib, to avoid intercostal arterial injury. In the authors' practice they always look for the sliding echogenic lung sign during inspiration to avoid potential injury to the lung. This technique is used when hepatic or splenic lesions are considered for biopsy (**Fig. 2**). This helps in determining a biopsy path to the lesion where no lung is visible in the field of view. They also use a high-frequency transducer with color Doppler to avoid vessels in the path of the needle biopsy. For targeted liver biopsies (**Fig. 3A–C**) they consider ultrasound as the tool of choice. With today's high-end equipment, including higher-frequency transducers with good penetration and improved hardware and software, one is able to see most of the hepatic lesions seen by CT or MR imaging. Most of the lesions initially missed by curvilinear probes are readily identifiable with higher-frequency linear or curvilinear probes. Lesions that are too high in the dome and those in the posterolateral aspect of the lateral segment of the left lobe are difficult to find because of shadowing from ribs and bowel. The use of fusion imaging makes it easier to identify smaller lesions for biopsy (**Fig. 3D**).

It has been advocated that a rind of normal hepatic parenchyma between the capsular puncture site and leading edge of the target lesion be present before attempting biopsy of peripheral hepatic lesions close to the capsule,[8] theoretically providing a tamponade mechanism for vascular tumors. Others have advocated the use of gel foam injection into the tract as the biopsy needle is withdrawn.[9] For severely coagulopathic patients requiring random liver biopsy, the transjugular route remains the method of choice.[10] The classic teaching is that ascites increases the risk of post-biopsy hemorrhage, because of a lack of tissue tamponade at the capsular puncture site. There are no data to support this claim, and there are data showing that perihepatic ascites does not affect the minor or major complication rate of hepatic biopsy.[11] Traversal of the portal and hepatic veins should be avoided, although this may not always be possible. Traversal of the hepatic arteries, especially centrally, should be avoided at all costs.[12]

Percutaneous random liver biopsy is one of the most common image-guided procedures in the abdomen. It is essential for histologic staging of chronic liver disease, and is also helpful for monitoring therapeutic effects of medical regimens.[13] This has been performed successfully without image guidance (blind), but has been shown to result in a higher complication rate.[14] The image-guided approach has been shown to be safe and effective in producing diagnostic core specimens.[15] For "random" core biopsies, the left hepatic lobe is the preferred target at the authors' institution, because it avoids the pleura and is usually better tolerated by the patient (**Fig. 4**). Although some have suggested that specimens from the right lobe may yield a more accurate histologic depiction of liver pathology, an autopsy study by Frankel and colleagues[16] demonstrated that no single site predicted pathologic findings better than any other site. Moreover, this group and others[17] have found that the right and left lobes were equal in providing diagnostic information. At the authors' institution, two 18-gauge cores nearly always yield adequate diagnostic results. The reader should, however, communicate with the pathologists at his or her institution to choose the appropriate biopsy device and size.

Targeted biopsies are also extremely common, especially at medical centers with large oncology practices. Very high success rates should be expected, assuming that the lesion is visible sonographically. One situation does warrant specific mention. Many tumors may be centrally necrotic, in which case the biopsy should be directed to the periphery of the lesion. This should be considered if a centrally placed needle fails to yield adequate cellular material.

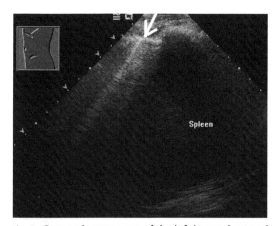

Fig. 2. Gray-scale sonogram of the left lower chest and spleen. A longitudinal image of the base of the left lung and the spleen is obtained before placement of a drainage catheter in the spleen using an intercostal approach. The ultrasound comet tail artifact (*arrow*) arising from the lung-wall interface is identified during respiration (sliding lung). This important sonographic sign helps avoid injury to the lung by selecting a different acoustic window to the splenic abscess.

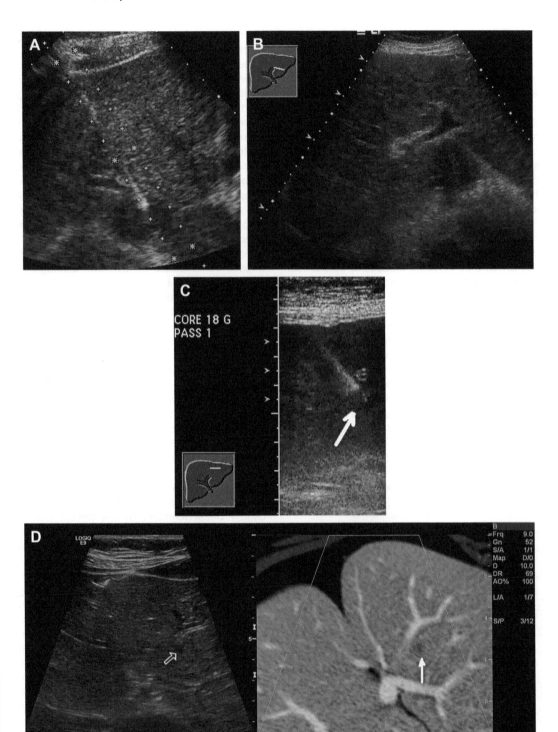

Fig. 3. Biopsy of different hepatic lesions. (*A*) Hepatocellular carcinoma. Sonogram showing a biopsy of a small hypoechoic lesion that was incidentally identified during renal ultrasound in this patient with known hepatitis C. (*B*) Diffuse melanoma metastases. Gray-scale sonogram of the liver obtained using a 4-MHz curvilinear probe showing multiple small hypoechoic lesions scattered through both the right and left lobes of the liver. (*C*) Same patient as in B. Use of high-resolution linear probe helps better localize a specific small lesion (*arrow*) for purposes of biopsy. (*D*) Fusion imaging. Suspected sarcoma metastasis. The combined ultrasound-CT image demonstrates that the small hypoechoic lesion behind the left portal vein is a metastatic focus, which correlates well with the CT scan. CT image (*solid arrow*). Ultrasound image (*open arrow*).

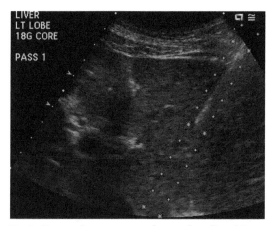

Fig. 4. Gray-scale sonogram of a random liver biopsy for persistent abnormal liver function test. The 18-gauge core biopsy is well seen in the lateral segment of the left lobe.

Pyogenic liver abscesses have been successfully treated with percutaneous aspiration or catheter drainage with sonographic guidance, in conjunction with antimicrobial therapy (Fig. 5).[18,19] Amebic abscesses have also been percutaneously aspirated, but data have shown that up to 90% of patients respond to metronidazole alone.[20] Rajak and colleagues[21] showed that catheter drainage was superior to aspiration only in a group of patients with both pyogenic and amebic abscesses. Although intraperitoneal amebic abscess rupture has traditionally carried with it a high mortality rate, Baijal and colleagues[22] achieved a 100% survival rate in 13 such patients, using percutaneous drainage with sonographic guidance.

Optimally, a puncture location allowing a normal rind of parenchyma is recommended, to minimize the potential chance of seeding into the peritoneal space. A liver abscess of less than 5 cm in size can be successfully treated with conservative therapy. An exception to this rule is an abscess located in the left lobe and close to the pericardium. Because of possible rupture into the pericardium these abscesses are usually drained regardless of size.

In addition to therapeutic abscess drainage, ultrasound can also aid in the placement of probes and needles for thermal ablation of hepatic tumors (Fig. 6). Multiple studies have reported the benefits of thermal ablation with sonographic guidance, including data from liver metastases[23] and hepatocellular carcinoma.[24,25] Sonography can also provide excellent real-time guidance for sclerotherapy of symptomatic hepatic cysts. Cyst aspiration followed by instillation of 95% to 96% ethanol in varying volumes has shown itself to be an effective therapy for symptomatic hepatic cysts, achieving volume reductions of 92.4% to 95%.[26,27] Before ethanol, injection of contrast under fluoroscopy or CT is recommended to exclude communication with the biliary tree or peritoneum.[28]

A novel use of ultrasound is for placement of "localization" coils into liver metastases before chemotherapy. There are data suggesting that microscopic viable tumor remains in hepatic sites of disease despite "complete" resolution by imaging, suggesting a therapeutic role for subsequent metastasectomy.[29] In cases such as this, the surgeon often cannot locate the microscopic focus at the time of resection. A vascular coil at

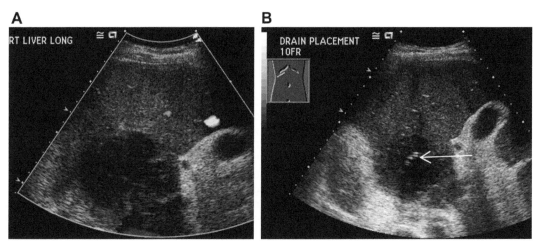

Fig. 5. (A) Gray-scale image demonstrates a relatively large cystic structure with debris seen in the right lobe of the liver. (B) Gray-scale sonogram showing a pigtail catheter (arrow) within the abscess cavity using the trocar technique.

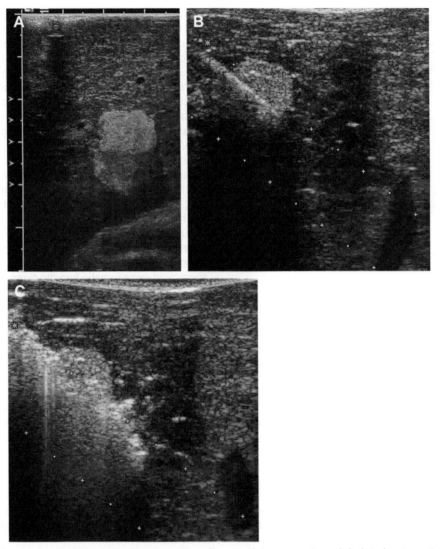

Fig. 6. (A) Gray-scale sonogram during intraoperative ultrasound demonstrating a lobulated metastatic echogenic mass in the liver from colon cancer. (B) A microwave ablation probe is placed within the mass. (C) The formation of the echogenic ball as a result of ablation is well appreciated with ultrasound. The mass is no longer appreciated.

the site can be localized with intraoperative ultrasound, allowing complete resection of the residual tumor (**Fig. 7**).

GALLBLADDER

Ultrasound is the ideal image guidance for cholecystic interventions, both diagnostic and therapeutic. In cases of gallbladder malignancy, percutaneous FNA with ultrasound guidance has been shown to be safe and effective, with a diagnostic accuracy of up to 95%.[30,31] Ultrasound-guided FNA has also shown promise in the diagnosis of xanthogranulomatous cholecystitis, although coexistent carcinoma cannot be entirely

excluded.[32] In addition, ultrasound is also the image guidance of choice for percutaneous cholecystostomy, usually performed for acute cholecystitis, and for malignant obstruction in patients who are not otherwise surgical candidates.[33] Both the transperitoneal and transhepatic (by the "bare area" of the gallbladder) routes have been described, although the transhepatic route is generally favored to minimize the risk of bile peritonitis or inadvertent colonic perforation.[18] The catheter must remain in place for at least 14 days, so that a mature epithelialized tract can form along the catheter. It is also recommended that a cholangiogram be performed before catheter removal, to ensure patency of the cystic and common bile

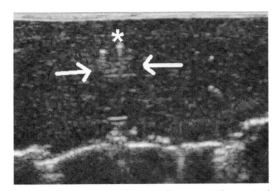

Fig. 7. Intraoperative ultrasound image of resected liver specimen from a patient with colon cancer metastasis treated with chemotherapy showing a small echogenic lesion (*between arrows*) in the center of the specimen reflecting residual tumor. Note the two small highly echogenic foci with comet tail artifact (*) representing a small coil that was placed before chemotherapy. The pathology result of this specimen was positive for tumor with negative margins.

ducts. The tract can also be injected after catheter removal, confirming a mature tract without leakage.[33] The most common complications encountered are hemorrhage (1.6%–2.2%) and bile leak or peritonitis (2.4%–4.4%), although pericholecystic abscess can also occur (**Fig. 8**).[33]

KIDNEY AND RETROPERITONEUM

Ultrasound-guided renal intervention is perhaps second only to liver intervention in overall frequency. The native kidneys are almost always well visualized sonographically, making this modality quite useful for diagnostic and therapeutic intervention. Much like the liver, there can be significant respiratory motion, necessitating real-time guidance. Both retroperitoneal (posterior) and peritoneal (anterior) approaches can be used. The posterior approach is preferred, because there are usually no intervening visceral structures. On occasion, however, the posterior approach may not be possible because of such conditions as hepatosplenomegaly or large patient size. In these cases an anterior approach can be attempted (**Fig. 9**). For random biopsies in the setting of suspected renal parenchymal disease, a posterior subcostal approach can usually be achieved to access the lower pole. For targeted intervention, an intercostal approach may be required. This approach limits the radiologist to a small acoustic window, in which case the small "footprint" of a vector probe can be useful.

The most common native renal intervention is cortical biopsy for "parenchymal disease." Core biopsy with sonographic guidance has been shown to yield diagnostic tissue specimens at a rate of up to 99% in adults[34] and 95% in children.[35] In a large prospective study in which patients underwent 14-gauge core renal biopsies,[36] a similar high diagnostic yield was noted. The minor (not requiring further intervention) complication rate was 9.5% and the major complication rate was 2.7%. Complications included perirenal hematoma (**Fig. 10**), AVF, hematuria, subcutaneous hematoma, and urinoma. Recommendations for postbiopsy observation times vary. Some research shows that a 6-hour

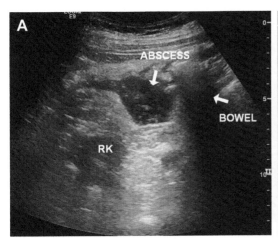
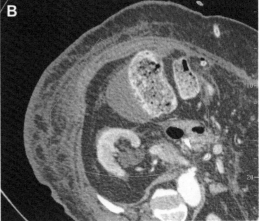

Fig. 8. (*A, B*) Fused ultrasound-CT image of an abdominal abscess following cholecystostomy for acute cholecystitis. The combined ultrasound-CT image nicely identifies the anatomic relation of the bowel to the abscess. The shadowing from the bowel is well correlated with the image from the CT. This makes visualization of the anatomy and abscess easy, an advantage fusion imaging can offer for interloop fluid collections.

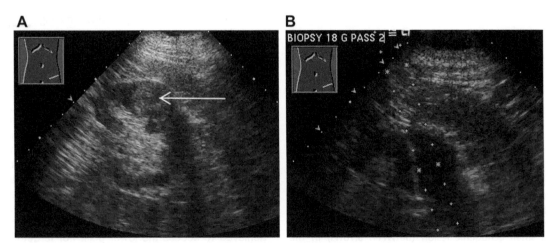

Fig. 9. (A) Sonogram showing a mass (*arrow*) in the left kidney suspicious for renal cell carcinoma. This mass was not seen from a posterior approach. (B) A biopsy from the anterior approach was completed successfully.

observation for outpatients is sufficient,[37] whereas others have shown that up to 33% of complications manifest themselves only after 8 hours.[38] The risk of bleeding does increase with worsening levels of renal insufficiency; poorly controlled hypertension has also been implicated as a risk factor for bleeding.[38]

Percutaneous core biopsies are essential in the management of renal transplant patients. Biopsy results are not only critical in treatment planning for graft dysfunction, but also for revealing subclinical rejection by surveillance, or "protocol" biopsies. There are data supporting the theory that early recognition of subclinical rejection can lead to therapies that improve long-term graft function.[39] In contradistinction to the native kidneys,

transplants are more superficial and have no respiratory motion, enhancing sonographic visualization. The polar cortex is the optimal target site, away from the central sinus complex and its vessels. The lower pole is preferable, because there is usually less subjacent bowel. Because of a higher concentration of cortex, this results in higher diagnostic yields. This approach also decreases the likelihood of hemorrhage, because it has been shown that the risk of hemorrhage is significantly higher if at least one core contains mostly medulla.[40] A lateral approach often approximates an avascular plane (Brödel's line) between the anterior and posterior divisions of the renal artery. The use of color Doppler in biopsy planning is also crucial, because superficial

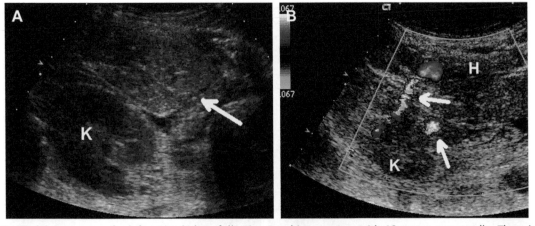

Fig. 10. (A) Sonogram of a left native kidney following two biopsy passes with 16-gauge core needle. There is a large hematoma (*arrow*) that formed anterior to the kidney immediately after the procedure was completed. k, kidney. (B) Color Doppler sonogram demonstrates active bleeding from two different sites presumably at each biopsy site (*arrows*). K, kidney; H, hematoma. Conservative measures failed to stop the bleeding, and subsequently the patient was treated with arterial embolization. The patient made a full recovery.

vessels, such as the circumflex iliac, and large intrarenal arteries can be avoided. Certain conditions, such as cortical atrophy or pre-existing AVFs from previous biopsies, can sometimes necessitate needle placement away from the polar regions. In these circumstances, a longitudinal oblique approach from the inferior pole can be useful, with a needle trajectory into the lateral cortex (**Fig. 11**). An upper pole transverse approach may also be possible, although care should be taken to avoid bowel.

Peritransplant fluid collections are quite common, occurring in 36% to 51% of patients.[41–43] Symptomatic collections or those temporally associated with rejection episodes can easily be accessed under sonographic guidance. Commonly encountered entities include seromas, hematomas, and lymphoceles, with abscesses and urinomas being less common.[41,42] The timeframe and sonographic features of the collections can often suggest the diagnosis (**Table 1**). Seromas, lymphoceles, and abscesses can all be accessed easily for catheter drainage. Trocar technique is usually successful, although postoperative fibrous tissue can sometimes impede catheter passage, in which case a Seldinger technique with serial dilation is usually successful. Percutaneous aspiration or drainage is often effective for lymphoceles,[44] and some have advocated this as a first line of therapy.[45] In cases of persistent lymphatic output, sclerotherapy can be attempted. Akhan and colleagues[46] demonstrated a 92% success rate with percutaneous transcatheter ethanol sclerotherapy in postoperative lymphoceles. Encouragingly, two of three patients in

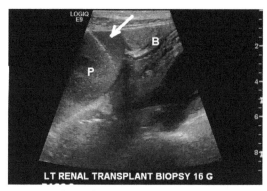

Fig. 11. High-resolution gray-scale sonogram with virtual convex. A 16-gauge core biopsy needle is shown in the lower pole of a transplant kidney (*arrow*) which is in a longitudinal orientation. The advantage of a high-resolution transducer (9–15 MHz) is that it provides excellent anatomic detail at the abdominal wall kidney interface. The pyramids (P) are also well appreciated and can be easily avoided. B, bowel.

their series who initially failed catheter drainage subsequently responded to sclerotherapy.

There is no universal consensus on the proper size of core biopsy device. A small prospective study has examined diagnostic efficacy and complication rates using 18-, 16-, and 14-gauge spring-loaded core devices.[47] No significant difference in complication rate was found between them, and the larger specimens yielded more glomeruli. The 14-gauge device did, however, result in significantly more pain at the time of biopsy. At the authors' institution, two 16-gauge specimens obtain a very high diagnostic yield, and are well tolerated by patients. The core specimens are immediately examined under light microscopy by the pathologist, to ensure adequacy. A clinician's own choice of needle size should, however, always be based on a mutual decision reached between him or her and the interpreting pathologist.

As compared with native kidney biopsies, transplant biopsies have been shown to have a lower overall complication rate. In a study in which both native and transplant kidneys underwent core biopsy, the overall complication rate for renal allografts was 8.7% compared with 19.4% for native kidneys, although the major complication rate was similar (2.9% and 2.4%, respectively).[36] The major difference was a higher minor complication rate for native kidneys. In a large series of patients, Schwarz and colleagues[48] reported an overall complication rate of 15% (gross hematuria, 3.2%; perirenal hematoma, 3.1%; AVF, 8.3%). They did note that 77% of AVFs resolved spontaneously. Hemodynamic significance was suspected by color Doppler in 2.1% of cases, although all of the patients with AVFs remained asymptomatic without any elevation of serum creatinine. Ultrasound including color and power Doppler plays a vital role in identifying early and late signs of biopsy complications (**Fig. 12**). The authors do not routinely perform postprocedure scans to look for complications, but if an abnormality is seen between passes, continued close monitoring is provided. The patients are kept for 4 hours after the procedure and monitored for hemodynamic changes. A complete blood count an hour before discharge is also obtained.

Traditionally, many have shied away from percutaneous biopsy of renal masses because of a fear of tumor seeding of the needle tract. The rate of seeding has likely been overstated, because no cases have been reported in the last 10 years.[49] Indeed, percutaneous biopsy has been shown to be a safe and accurate method for evaluating renal masses.[50–52] In the setting of a known extrarenal primary tumor or lymphoma, biopsy can be useful

Table 1
Common peritransplant fluid collections

	Time Frame	Sonographic Features	Intervention
Hematoma/seroma	Immediate postoperative period	Acute hematomas are hyperechoic and complex; resolving hematomas become progressively more hypoechoic and often anechoic (cystic); common	Usually none needed, unless to differentiate from abscess; usually not well drained with a catheter
Lymphocele	Usually 4–8 wk after surgery	Cystic collection usually with multiple septations	Catheter drainage is often curative, although sclerotherapy may be required in resistant cases
Abscess	Early postoperative period	Complex fluid collection, usually in the setting of fever and elevated white blood cell count; may display surrounding hyperemia on color Doppler; rare	Catheter drainage is required and usually beneficial
Urinoma	Early postoperative period	Usually caused by ischemic necrosis of the distal ureter or ureterovesicle anastomotic leak; relatively simple fluid collection; rare	Aspiration with evaluation of creatinine level can be confirmatory, although renal scintigraphy usually diagnostic

to differentiate renal cell carcinoma from these two entities. It can also be useful for confirmation of renal cell carcinoma in small solid lesions and indeterminate cystic masses, and a confirmatory role before percutaneous thermal ablation.[53] FNA with or without flow cytometry is often sufficient, although core specimens can be additive. Hunter and colleagues,[54] for example, showed that core biopsy had a higher diagnostic yield than FNA for the diagnosis of lymphoma, whereas Heilbrun and colleagues[49] noted that FNA had a higher sensitivity for renal neoplasm.

Ultrasound can also provide guidance for therapeutic intervention. Percutaneous drainage of renal, perirenal, and psoas abscesses has been shown to be efficacious.[55,56] Because of their retroperitoneal location, these structures are usually well visualized sonographically. Transient bacteremia is a not uncommon complication of catheter placement, and the radiologist should monitor the patient closely for signs of sepsis. Aspiration of indeterminate renal masses can also differentiate between neoplastic and benign conditions (**Fig. 13**). In addition, ultrasound has been useful as a guidance method for percutaneous thermal ablation of renal cell carcinoma.[57]

Sonographic guidance has been used for sclerotherapy of symptomatic renal cysts. Decreased patient pain has been noted with cyst aspiration followed by the injection of 95% to 99% ethanol.[58,59] Before ethanol, injection of contrast under fluoroscopy or CT is recommended to exclude communication with the collecting system.[28]

OMENTUM AND PERITONEUM

Paracentesis is one of the most common abdominal interventions performed under sonographic guidance. It can serve a diagnostic role, such as evaluation for malignant ascites or spontaneous bacterial peritonitis, and a therapeutic role in cases of tense ascites. Puncture into the largest fluid pocket is usually straightforward, although caution should be used to avoid the epigastric artery or abdominal wall portosystemic collaterals. The authors perform ultrasound guidance only in cases with small volume for diagnostic purposes (**Fig. 14**). Complications reported include inferior epigastric arterial injury, bowel perforation, hypotension, and hemorrhage after large-volume paracentesis. If a large volume of fluid (>5 L) is

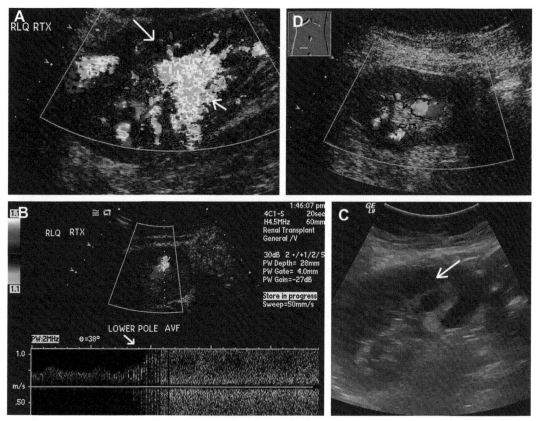

Fig. 12. Vascular complications of kidney transplant biopsy. (*A*) Arteriovenous fistula. Color Doppler sonogram showing characteristic color artifact from tissue reverberations (between *arrows*). (*B*) Spectral Doppler sonogram of the arteriovenous fistula with typical arterial venous mixing waveform (*arrow*). (*C*) Intrarenal pseudoaneurysm. The gray-scale image shows what resembles calyceal dilatation (*arrow*) in the lower pole of kidney transplant. (*D*) Color Doppler sonogram of the same kidney demonstrates the characteristic Ying-Yang sign indicating that what looks like calyceal dilation is actually an arterial pseudoaneurysm.

removed, one should be aware of the possibility of postparacentesis circulatory dysfunction. This manifests as hypotension, azotemia, hyponatremia, and an increase in plasma renin activity.[18] Albumin (8 g/L of removed fluid) has been the standard treatment method,[60] although there is evidence that terlipressin is as effective in preventing hemodynamic changes.[61]

Although many assume that CT is the easiest guidance method for omental and extravisceral peritoneal biopsies, the opposite often proves true. For example, Gottlieb and colleagues[62] demonstrated successful needle placement in a series of 52 patients, and demonstrated the added benefit of reduced distance to the target compared with CT. Recent CT scans can also act as a guide. The hesitation to use ultrasound likely stems from a fear of inadvertent bowel perforation, but this has been shown to be an uncommon complication, even with 18-gauge cutting needles.[63] The use of firm pressure with the transducer is important for two reasons. First,

it decreases the distance to target. Second, it can help fixate otherwise mobile omental lesions so that needle penetration can be achieved. Omental biopsy under sonographic guidance has also recently been shown to be useful in tracing the origin of unclear ascites in the setting of omental thickening, showing high sensitivity and specificity (95.6% and 92.9%, respectively) for differentiating between benign and malignant ascites (**Fig. 15**).[64]

Sonography also proves useful for accessing loculated peritoneal fluid collections, both for percutaneous sampling and therapeutic catheter drainage. Primary indications for drainage include treatment of sepsis related to an infected collection and alleviation of symptoms caused by mass effect.[55] Percutaneous drainage has had a major impact on the treatment of intra-abdominal infection over the past two decades.[65] The efficacy of percutaneous approaches has been shown, because Akinci and colleagues[66] demonstrated an overall success rate of 91% in a series of 255

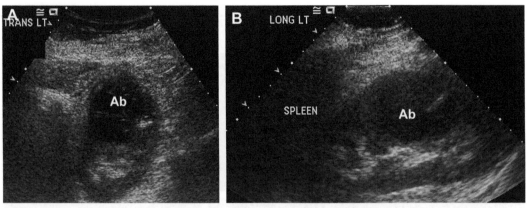

Fig. 13. (*A, B*) Renal abscess. Young woman with flank pain, fever, and abnormal urine test. Ultrasound shows large cystic lesion (Ab) in the interpolar region of the left kidney with internal debris consistent with abscess.

patients. After catheter placement, regular flushes with sterile saline are crucial to maintain catheter patency. Most abscesses should have gradually diminishing output. If catheter output increases or remains greater than 100 mL per 24 hours for more than 4 days after placement, a gastrointestinal fistula should be suspected.[18] Sinography can then confirm communication with bowel. Although percutaneous drainage has a high success rate overall, there are some data suggesting lower success rates in collections containing yeast.[65] Multilocular collections can also be problematic, although urokinase irrigation has been recommended.[28] The septations themselves are often more apparent on ultrasound as compared with CT, which can help in predicting efficacy.

Lymphoceles are typically well visualized sonographically. Using sonographic guidance, Akhan and colleagues[46] aspirated 62 pelvic lymphoceles under sonographic guidance, replacing half the volume with absolute ethanol, achieving an initial treatment success rate of 91%. The cavities were injected with contrast under fluoroscopy before ethanol ablation, to exclude extravasation into the peritoneum, which is a contraindication.

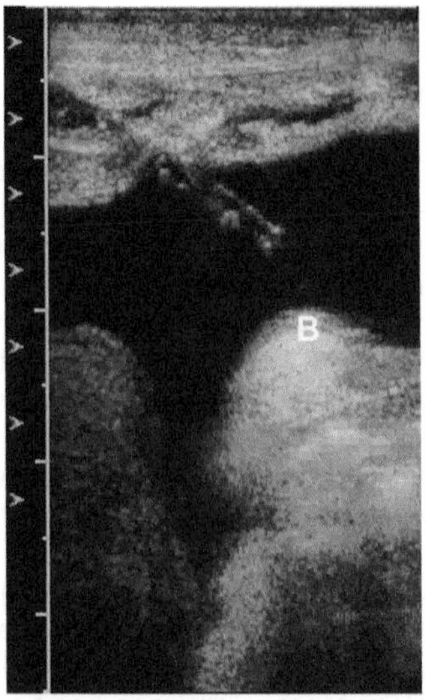

PANCREAS

Today, ultrasound-guided biopsy of the pancreas is almost exclusively performed under endoscopic ultrasound guidance. In the past decade, this trend has been adopted by clinicians because of better visualization of lesions as a result of better image resolution and close proximity of the pancreas to the stomach. Despite this trend of change the diagnostic rates and sensitivities for endoscopic ultrasound and transabdominal biopsies have been shown to be equal.[67] There are a number of complications associated with pancreatic biopsies, with 3% of all biopsies resulting in severe acute pancreatitis.[68]

Percutaneous core biopsies are essential for proper management of pancreatic allograft recipients, both in the setting of graft dysfunction[69] and surveillance.[70] As opposed to renal allograft biopsies, pancreatic allograft biopsies are much more challenging. Despite some form of fixation to the ventral abdominal wall, much of the graft is often obscured by closely opposed small bowel. There is usually only a small acoustic window through which to visualize the graft and pass the biopsy needle. These difficulties are reflected in a review

Fig. 14. Paracentesis. Patient with low-volume ascites. Gray-scale image obtained with high-resolution linear probe showing the Yueh needle catheter entering ascitic fluid. Note close proximity of bowel loops (B) to the catheter. This is one situation where such a procedure is safely performed under ultrasound guidance.

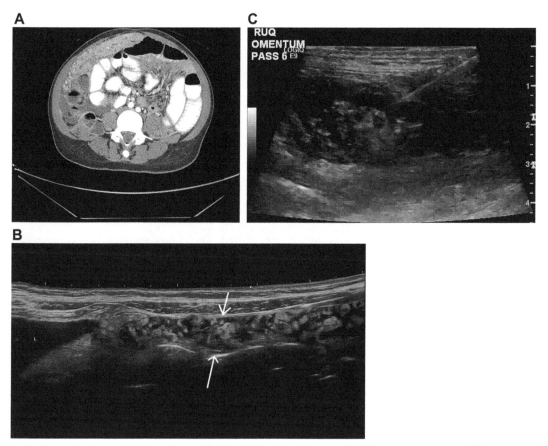

Fig. 15. Omental tuberculosis in patient with HIV-AIDS and weight loss. (*A*) CT scan demonstrates diffuse omental thickening and caking. Concern for malignancy was raised by the clinical team. (*B*) Gray-scale image using extended field of view nicely demonstrates the extensive omental thickening (between *arrows*) extending to the tip of the left lobe or the liver. (*C*) Fine-needle aspiration of the omentum showed no evidence of malignancy; instead, multiple granulomas suspicious for tuberculosis were seen.

of 120 biopsies,[71] which showed that even with ultrasound guidance, 15% of the biopsies contained no pancreatic tissue. Nondiagnostic specimens contained fat and small bowel, and 9% of the patients had biochemical pancreatitis, although they remained asymptomatic. In these cases, use of a high-frequency linear transducer is essential, because it provides better visualization of interposed bowel (**Fig. 16**). The free-hand technique provides greater flexibility, but requires operator experience. Needle guides are widely available, and can potentially shorten the procedure time.

Ultrasound is useful for guiding interventions in the setting of pancreatitis. Percutaneous drainage of infected necrosis, abscess, and pancreatic pseudocyst has been well described (**Fig. 17**).[72] Ultrasound can be used so long as bowel gas does not obscure the underlying collections. The transgastric approach has been described,[73] but the catheter must often be left for 2 weeks or

greater to create an epithelialized tract.[55] Sinography should be performed as follow-up prior to catheter removal to assess for cavity size, pancreatic ductal communication, and cystenteric fistula.[74]

SPLEEN AND LYMPH NODES

The spleen is usually well visualized sonographically, and ultrasound is a valuable guidance method for percutaneous intervention. Percutaneous sampling is especially important for characterizing focal lesions, because imaging characteristics alone are usually nonspecific (**Fig. 18**). The spleen can also act as an acoustic window for the biopsy of deep peritoneal lesions (**Fig. 19**). Either subcostal or intercostal approaches can be used, depending on the location of the lesion in the spleen. The intercostal approach has a risk of pneumothorax and bleeding from injury to a intercostal artery. One patient in a series of

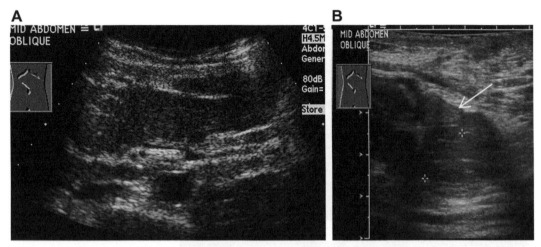

Fig. 16. Pancreatic transplant biopsy performed to rule out rejection. (*A*) A curvilinear ultrasound image demonstrates the pancreatic transplant clearly. (*B*) Same pancreas imaged with high-resolution linear probe identifies unsuspected loop of small bowel (*arrow*) between the pancreas and the abdominal wall. Such information can easily be missed if one has attempted to perform the biopsy with the lower-frequency curvilinear probe. With the use of the high-resolution probe one manages to see the bowel and avoid it during the biopsy.

50 had a pneumothorax,[75] although others have not reported this complication. Although there is often reluctance to biopsy the spleen because of concerns over hemorrhage, there are actually data suggesting that percutaneous biopsy is safe and efficacious. Kang and colleagues[76] performed FNA biopsies, aspiration, and catheter drainages in 89 patients. No major complications were noted. Another series of 32 patients undergoing FNA for focal splenic lesions had only one case of hemorrhage, and it did not require transfusion.[77] In another series of 160 patients undergoing FNA, no major complications were encountered and the authors reported a sensitivity of 98% and positive predictive value of 99%.[78] Core biopsy with 18-gauge needles has also been shown to be safe and effective, both in adults[79] and children.[80]

Percutaneous drainage of splenic abscesses has also been described, with a high success rate (**Fig. 20**),[76,81] although the total number of patients reported is quite small. One patient out of a series of seven required splenectomy because of hemorrhage following catheter insertion.[81]

Given the relatively limited data in the literature regarding splenic intervention, it seems that the risk of hemorrhage is perhaps not significantly greater in comparison with the other solid organs.

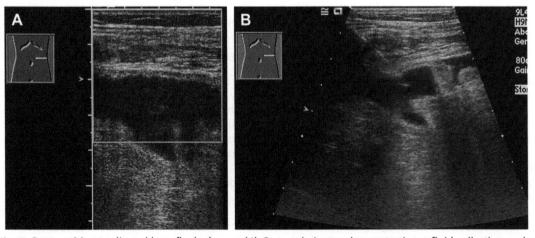

Fig. 17. Pancreatitis complicated by a flank abscess. (*A*) Gray-scale image demonstrating a fluid collection under the abdominal wall in the left flank. (*B*) Sonogram showing pigtail catheter being advanced into abscess.

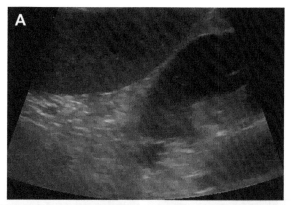

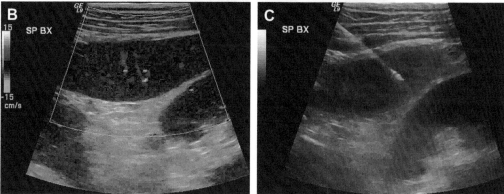

Fig. 18. Splenic granulomas. Young male patient with history of HIV presented with splenomegaly. CT scan (not shown) was positive for multiple small low-attenuation lesions in the spleen with splenomegaly. Ultrasound-guided biopsy was requested to exclude lymphoma. (*A*) Gray-scale sonogram demonstrates multiple hypoechoic lesions in the spleen. (*B*) Color Doppler image of the spleen shows no evidence of increased vascularity to any of the splenic lesions. (*C*) Fine-needle aspiration biopsy of the largest lesion using a subcostal approach showed multiple granulomas.

When suspicious similar lesions are present in both the spleen and another organ, such as the liver, consideration for biopsy should be given to the liver.

Peritoneal and retroperitoneal lymphadenopathy is a common indication for percutaneous abdominal biopsies. There is ample evidence that sonography provides safe and effective needle

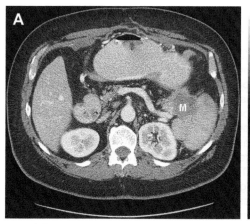

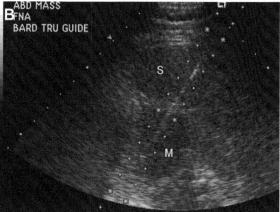

Fig. 19. (*A*) CT scan with a low-attenuation mass medial to the spleen. The mass (M) seems to grow into the spleen. (*B*) Gray-scale image of the mass (M), which was biopsied through the spleen (S).

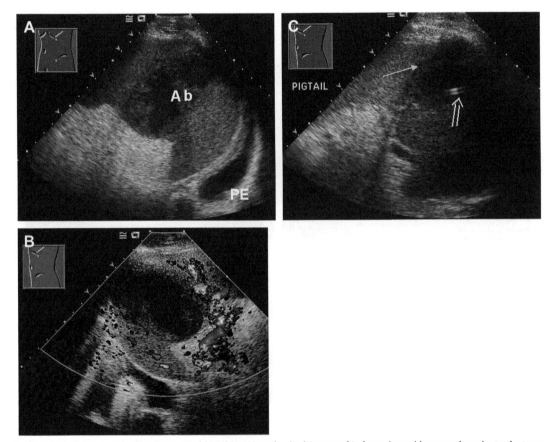

Fig. 20. Splenic abscesses. This 60-year-old male patient had a history of infected total knee arthroplasty that progressed to endocarditis, septicemia, and multiple splenic abscesses. He was gravely ill and not fit for surgery. We were asked to drain the largest splenic abscess in the ICU. (*A*) Gray-scale image. A large splenic abscess is seen (Ab). There is also a small left-sided pleural effusion (PE). (*B*) Color Doppler sonogram helps identify the vascular structures so that they can be avoided during the procedure. (*C*) Using the Seldinger technique a pigtail catheter (*open arrow*) was placed into the abscess (*solid arrow*).

guidance for nodal biopsies.[82–84] In a series of 102 patients undergoing FNA, Gupta and colleagues[82] showed a diagnostic rate of 85% with no major or minor complications, even in cases of a transhepatic route and despite the fact that no particular care was taken to avoid traversal of bowel. The advantages of sonographic guidance over CT have been demonstrated, including multiplanar capability, decreased distance to target of up to 50%, and real-time visualization of the needle pass, minimizing potential contamination from adjacent tissues.[84] FNA of abdominal lymphadenopathy in HIV patients under sonographic guidance has also been shown to be efficacious and safe, with a diagnostic yield rate of 87.5%.[85]

ABDOMINAL WALL AND SUPERFICIAL STRUCTURES

Given their superficial location, fluid collections and masses in the abdominal wall are particularly

well suited to ultrasound-guided intervention. Masses can also be localized with a wire before surgical resection (**Fig. 21**), similar to needle localization before lumpectomy.

SUMMARY

Ultrasound is a valuable tool for both diagnostic and therapeutic percutaneous applications in the abdomen. Numerous advantages over CT include faster procedure times, real-time needle visualization, decreased cost, and a lack of ionizing radiation. Newer technology, such as image fusion, has allowed the radiologist to simultaneously use the advantages of two modalities, ultrasound and CT or MR imaging, to localize lesions. The use of high-resolution probes and color Doppler to assess the superficial anatomy before any interventional procedure is strongly advocated. Such implementation prevents many of the inadvertently injured vascular structures or nonvisualized loops

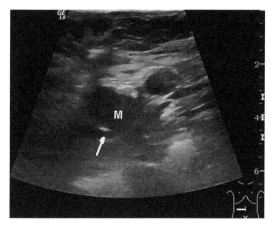

Fig. 21. Recurrent abdominal wall metastasis from colon cancer following resection of primary tumor. This patient has had one prior surgery for the same reason. Because of extensive adhesions at the site of prior surgery the authors were asked to place a wire into the lesion to help in localizing the mass for resection. Echogenic wire (*arrow*) was placed under ultrasound guidance into the mass (M) on the morning of the surgery. Complete resection was achieved.

of small bowel stuck against the abdominal wall lying in the path of the biopsy needle.

There is no doubt that as the bodies in the United States are becoming more aware of the risks of radiation exposure to the population from CT, ultrasound will regain its position as the first diagnostic imaging modality, and may become the imaging modality of choice for all interventions.

REFERENCES

1. Dodd GD III, Esola CC, Memel DS, et al. Sonography: the undiscovered jewel of interventional radiology. Radiographics 1996;16(6):1271–88.
2. Sheafor DH, Paulson EK, Simmons CM, et al. Abdominal percutaneous interventional procedures: comparison of CT and US guidance. Radiology 1998;207(3):705–10.
3. Kliewer MA, Sheafor DH, Paulson EK, et al. Percutaneous liver biopsy: a cost-benefit analysis comparing sonographic and CT guidance. AJR Am J Roentgenol 1999;173(5):1199–202.
4. Hall EJ, Brenner DJ. Cancer risks from diagnostic radiology. Br J Radiol 2008;81(965):362–78.
5. O'Connell AM, Keeling F, Given M, et al. Fine-needle Tru-Cut biopsy versus fine-needle aspiration cytology with ultrasound guidance in the abdomen. J Med Imaging Radiat Oncol 2008;52(3):231–6.
6. Hugosson CO, Nyman RS, Cappelen-Smith JM, et al. Ultrasound-guided biopsy of abdominal and pelvic lesions in children: a comparison between fine needle aspiration and 1.2 mm-needle core biopsy. Pediatr Radiol 1999;29(1):31–6.
7. Quinn SF, vanSonnenberg E, Casola G, et al. Interventional radiology in the spleen. Radiology 1986; 161:289–91.
8. Gupta S, Madoff DC. Image-guided percutaneous needle biopsy in cancer diagnosis and staging. Tech Vasc Interv Radiol 2007;10(2):88–101.
9. Hoffer FA. Liver biopsy methods for pediatric oncology patients. Pediatr Radiol 2000;30(7):481–8.
10. Senzolo M, Burra P, Cholongitas E, et al. The transjugular route: the key hole to the liver world. Dig Liver Dis 2007;39(2):105–16.
11. Little AF, Ferris JV, Dodd GD III, et al. Image-guided percutaneous hepatic biopsy: effect of ascites on the complication rate. Radiology 1996;199(1):79–83.
12. Winter TC, Lee FT Jr, Hinshaw JL. Ultrasound-guided biopsies in the abdomen and pelvis. Ultrasound Q 2008;24(1):45–68.
13. Spiezia S, Salvio A, Di Somma C, et al. The efficacy of liver biopsy under ultrasonographic guidance on an outpatient basis. Eur J Ultrasound 2002;15(3): 127–31.
14. Lindor KD, Bru C, Jorgensen RA, et al. The role of ultrasonography and automatic-needle biopsy in outpatient percutaneous liver biopsy. Hepatology 1996;23(5):1079–83.
15. Rivera-Sanfeliz G, Kinney TB, Rose SC, et al. Single-pass percutaneous liver biopsy for diffuse liver disease using an automated device: experience in 154 procedures. Cardiovasc Intervent Radiol 2005; 28(5):584–8.
16. Frankel WL, Tranovich JG, Salter L, et al. The optimal number of donor biopsy sites to evaluate liver histology for transplantation. Liver Transpl 2002; 8(11):1044–50.
17. Picciotto A, Ciravegna G, Lapertosa G, et al. One or two liver biopsies during laparoscopy? Hepatogastroenterology 1983;30(5):192–3.
18. Nakamoto DA, Haaga JR. Emergent ultrasound interventions. Radiol Clin North Am 2004;42(2):457–78.
19. Giorgio A, Tarantino L, Mariniello N, et al. Pyogenic liver abscesses: 13 years of experience in percutaneous needle aspiration with US guidance. Radiology 1995;195(1):122–4.
20. Weinke T, Grobusch MP, Güthoff W. Amebic liver abscess: rare need for percutaneous treatment modalities. Eur J Med Res 2002;7(1):25–9.
21. Rajak CL, Gupta S, Jain S, et al. Percutaneous treatment of liver abscesses: needle aspiration versus catheter drainage. AJR Am J Roentgenol 1998; 170(4):1035–9.
22. Baijal SS, Agarwal DK, Roy S, et al. Complex ruptured amebic liver abscesses: the role of percutaneous catheter drainage. Eur J Radiol 1995;20(1):65–7.
23. Hofer S, Oberholzer C, Beck S, et al. Ultrasound-guided radiofrequency ablation (RFA) for inoperable

gastrointestinal liver metastases. Ultraschall Med 2008;29(4):388–92.

24. Yan K, Chen MH, Yang W, et al. Radiofrequency ablation of hepatocellular carcinoma: long-term outcome and prognostic factors. Eur J Radiol 2008;67(2):336–47.

25. Hänsler J, Frieser M, Tietz V, et al. Percutaneous ultrasound-guided radiofrequency ablation (RFA) using saline-perfused (wet) needle electrodes for the treatment of hepatocellular carcinoma: long term experience. Ultraschall Med 2007;28(6): 604–11.

26. Zerem E, Imamović G, Omerović S. Percutaneous treatment of symptomatic non-parasitic benign liver cysts: single-session alcohol sclerotherapy versus prolonged catheter drainage with negative pressure. Eur Radiol 2008;18(2):400–6 [erratum in: Eur Radiol 2008;18(2):407].

27. Larssen TB, Rosendahl K, Horn A, et al. Single-session alcohol sclerotherapy in symptomatic benign hepatic cysts performed with a time of exposure to alcohol of 10 min: initial results. Eur Radiol 2003;13(12):2627–32.

28. Lohela P. Ultrasound-guided drainages and sclerotherapy. Eur Radiol 2002;12(2):288–95.

29. Benoist S, Brouquet A, Penna C, et al. Complete response of colorectal liver metastases after chemotherapy: does it mean cure? J Clin Oncol 2006;24: 3939–45.

30. Venkataramu NK, Sood BP, Gupta S, et al. Ultrasound-guided fine needle aspiration biopsy of gall bladder malignancies. Acta Radiol 1999;40(4):436–9.

31. Shukla VK, Pandey M, Kumar M, et al. Ultrasound-guided fine needle aspiration cytology of malignant gallbladder masses. Acta Cytol 1997;41(6):1654–8.

32. Krishnani N, Dhingra S, Kapoor S, et al. Cytopathologic diagnosis of xanthogranulomatous cholecystitis and coexistent lesions: a prospective study of 31 cases. Acta Cytol 2007;51(1):37–41.

33. Ginat D, Saad WE. Cholecystostomy and transcholecystic biliary access. Tech Vasc Interv Radiol 2008;11(1):2–13.

34. Tung KT, Downes MO, O'Donnell PJ. Renal biopsy in diffuse renal disease: experience with a 14-gauge automated biopsy gun. Clin Radiol 1992;46(2): 111–3.

35. Nammalwar BR, Vijayakumar M, Prahlad N. Experience of renal biopsy in children with nephrotic syndrome. Pediatr Nephrol 2006;21(2):286–8.

36. Preda A, Van Dijk LC, Van Oostaijen JA, et al. Complication rate and diagnostic yield of 515 consecutive ultrasound-guided biopsies of renal allografts and native kidneys using a 14-gauge Biopty gun. Eur Radiol 2003;13(3):527–30.

37. Lin WC, Yang Y, Wen YK, et al. Outpatient versus inpatient renal biopsy: a retrospective study. Clin Nephrol 2006;66(1):17–24.

38. Whittier WL, Korbet SM. Timing of complications in percutaneous renal biopsy. J Am Soc Nephrol 2004;15(1):142–7.

39. Rush D, Nickerson P, Gough J, et al. Beneficial effects of treatment of early subclinical rejection: a randomized study. J Am Soc Nephrol 1998; 9(11):2129–34.

40. Beckingham IJ, Nicholson ML, Bell PR. Analysis of factors associated with complications following renal transplant needle core biopsy. Br J Urol 1994;73(1):13–5.

41. Pollak R, Veremis SA, Maddux MS, et al. The natural history of and therapy for perirenal fluid collections following renal transplantation. J Urol 1988;140(4): 716–20.

42. Silver TM, Campbell D, Wicks JD, et al. Peritransplant fluid collections: ultrasound evaluation and clinical significance. Radiology 1981;138(1):145–51.

43. Khauli RB, Stoff JS, Lovewell T, et al. Post-transplant lymphoceles: a critical look into the risk factors, pathophysiology and management. J Urol 1993; 150(1):22–6.

44. White M, Mueller PR, Ferrucci JT Jr, et al. Percutaneous drainage of postoperative abdominal and pelvic lymphoceles. AJR Am J Roentgenol 1985; 145(5):1065–9.

45. Zietek Z, Sulikowski T, Tejchman K, et al. Lymphocele after kidney transplantation. Transplant Proc 2007;39(9):2744–7.

46. Akhan O, Karcaaltincaba M, Ozmen MN, et al. Percutaneous transcatheter ethanol sclerotherapy and catheter drainage of postoperative pelvic lymphoceles. Cardiovasc Intervent Radiol 2007;30(2):237–40.

47. Nicholson ML, Wheatley TJ, Doughman TM, et al. A prospective randomized trial of three different sizes of core-cutting needle for renal transplant biopsy. Kidney Int 2000;58(1):390–5.

48. Schwarz A, Hiss M, Gwinner W, et al. Course and relevance of arteriovenous fistulas after renal transplant biopsies. Am J Transplant 2008;8(4):826–31.

49. Heilbrun ME, Zagoria RJ, Garvin AJ, et al. CT-guided biopsy for the diagnosis of renal tumors before treatment with percutaneous ablation. AJR Am J Roentgenol 2007;188(6):1500–5.

50. Jaff A, Molinié V, Mellot F, et al. Evaluation of imaging-guided fine-needle percutaneous biopsy of renal masses. Eur Radiol 2005;15(8):1721–6.

51. Hara I, Miyake H, Hara S, et al. Role of percutaneous image-guided biopsy in the evaluation of renal masses. Urol Int 2001;67(3):199–202.

52. Schmidbauer J, Remzi M, Memarsadeghi M, et al. Diagnostic accuracy of computed tomography-guided percutaneous biopsy of renal masses. Eur Urol 2008;53(5):1003–11.

53. Silverman SG, Gan YU, Mortele KJ, et al. Renal masses in the adult patient: the role of percutaneous biopsy. Radiology 2006;240(1):6–22.

54. Hunter S, Samir A, Eisner B, et al. Diagnosis of renal lymphoma by percutaneous image guided biopsy: experience with 11 cases. J Urol 2006;176(5): 1952–6 [discussion: 1956].

55. Men S, Akhan O, Köroğlu M. Percutaneous drainage of abdominal abscess. Eur J Radiol 2002;43(3):204–18.

56. Dahniya MH, Hanna RM, Grexa E, et al. Percutaneous drainage of tuberculous iliopsoas abscesses under image guidance. Australas Radiol 1999;43(4):444–7.

57. Veltri A, Garetto I, Pagano E, et al. Percutaneous RF thermal ablation of renal tumors: is US guidance really less favorable than other imaging guidance techniques? Cardiovasc Intervent Radiol 2009;32(1):76–85.

58. Paananen I, Hellström P, Leinonen S, et al. Treatment of renal cysts with single-session percutaneous drainage and ethanol sclerotherapy: long-term outcome. Urology 2001;57(1):30–3.

59. Mohsen T, Gomha MA. Treatment of symptomatic simple renal cysts by percutaneous aspiration and ethanol sclerotherapy. BJU Int 2005;96(9):1369–72.

60. Velamati PG, Herlong HF. Treatment of refractory ascites. Curr Treat Options Gastroenterol 2006;9(6):530–7.

61. Lata J, Marecek Z, Fejfar T, et al. The efficacy of terlipressin in comparison with albumin in the prevention of circulatory changes after the paracentesis of tense ascites: a randomized multicentric study. Hepatogastroenterology 2007;54(79):1930–3.

62. Gottlieb RH, Tan R, Widjaja J, et al. Extravisceral masses in the peritoneal cavity: sonographically guided biopsies in 52 patients. AJR Am J Roentgenol 1998;171(3):697–701.

63. Ho LM, Thomas J, Fine SA, et al. Usefulness of sonographic guidance during percutaneous biopsy of mesenteric masses. AJR Am J Roentgenol 2003; 180(6):1563–6.

64. Que Y, Wang X, Liu Y, et al. Ultrasound-guided biopsy of greater omentum: an effective method to trace the origin of unclear ascites. Eur J Radiol 2008 March 5 (Epub ahead of print).

65. Cinat ME, Wilson SE, Din AM. Determinants for successful percutaneous image guided drainage of intra-abdominal abscess. Arch Surg 2002; 137(7):845–9.

66. Akinci D, Akhan O, Ozmen MN, et al. Percutaneous drainage of 300 intraperitoneal abscesses with long-term follow-up. Cardiovasc Intervent Radiol 2005; 28(6):744–50.

67. Erturk SM, Mortelé KJ, Tuncali K, et al. Fine-needle aspiration biopsy of solid pancreatic masses: comparison of CT and endoscopic sonography guidance. AJR Am J Roentgenol 2006;187(6):1531–5.

68. Mueller PR, Miketic LM, Simeone JF, et al. Severe acute pancreatitis after percutaneous biopsy of the pancreas. AJR Am J Roentgenol 1988;151(3):493–4.

69. Klassen DK, Weir MR, Cangro CB, et al. Pancreas allograft biopsy: safety of percutaneous biopsy-results of a large experience. Transplantation 2002;73(4):553–5.

70. Stratta RJ, Taylor RJ, Grune MT, et al. Experience with protocol biopsies after solitary pancreas transplantation. Transplantation 1995;60(12):1431–7.

71. Malek SK, Potdar S, Martin JA, et al. Percutaneous ultrasound-guided pancreas allograft biopsy: a single-center experience. Transplant Proc 2005; 37(10):4436–7.

72. Shankar S, vanSonnenberg E, Silverman SG, et al. Imaging and percutaneous management of acute complicated pancreatitis. Cardiovasc Intervent Radiol 2004;27(6):567–80.

73. Davies RP, Cox MR, Wilson TG, et al. Percutaneous cystogastrostomy with a new catheter for drainage of pancreatic pseudocysts and fluid collections. Cardiovasc Intervent Radiol 1996;19(2):128–31.

74. Neff R. Pancreatic pseudocysts and fluid collections: percutaneous approaches. Surg Clin North Am 2001;81(2):399–403, xii.

75. Caraway NP, Fanning CV. Use of fine needle aspiration biopsy in the evaluation of splenic lesions in a cancer center. Diagn Cytopathol 1997;16:312–6.

76. Kang M, Kalra N, Gulati M, et al. Image guided percutaneous splenic interventions. Eur J Radiol 2007;64(1):140–6.

77. Venkataramu NK, Gupta S, Sood BP, et al. Ultrasound guided fine needle aspiration biopsy of splenic lesions. Br J Radiol 1999;72(862):953–6.

78. Cavanna L, Lazzaro A, Vallisa D, et al. Role of image-guided fine-needle aspiration biopsy in the management of patients with splenic metastasis. World J Surg Oncol 2007;5:13.

79. Liang P, Gao Y, Wang Y, et al. US-guided percutaneous needle biopsy of the spleen using 18-gauge versus 21-gauge needles. J Clin Ultrasound 2007; 35(9):477–82.

80. Muraca S, Chait PG, Connolly BL, et al. US-guided core biopsy of the spleen in children. Radiology 2001;218(1):200–6.

81. Lucey BC, Boland GW, Maher MM, et al. Percutaneous nonvascular splenic intervention: a 10-year review. AJR Am J Roentgenol 2002;179(6):1591–6.

82. Gupta S, Rajak CL, Sood BP, et al. Sonographically guided fine needle aspiration biopsy of abdominal lymph nodes: experience in 102 patients. J Ultrasound Med 1999;18(2):135–9.

83. Fisher AJ, Paulson EK, Sheafor DH, et al. Small lymph nodes of the abdomen, pelvis, and retroperitoneum: usefulness of sonographically guided biopsy. Radiology 1997;205(1):185–90.

84. Memel DS, Dodd GD III, Esola CC. Efficacy of sonography as a guidance technique for biopsy of abdominal, pelvic, and retroperitoneal lymph nodes. AJR Am J Roentgenol 1996;167(4):957–62.

85. Veerapand P, Chotimanvijit R, Laohasrisakul N, et al. Percutaneous ultrasound-guided fine needle aspiration of abdominal lymphadenopathy in AIDS patients. J Med Assoc Thai 2004;87(4):400–4.

Ultrasound-Guided Kidney Biopsies

Yueh Z. Lee, MD, PhD[a], JulieAnne McGregor, MD[b],
Wui K. Chong, MBBS, MRCP, FRCR[a],*

KEYWORDS

- Kidneys • Biopsy • Ultrasound • Guidance
- Complications • Transplant

The purpose of nontargeted renal biopsy is to obtain a sample of renal cortex (and sometimes medulla) for tissue diagnosis of renal parenchymal disease. Imaging guidance is used in most instances, and ultrasound is the modality of choice because it is real time, quick, and easy to use. Acute renal injury and chronic renal injury are major causes of morbidity, mortality, and health care expenditure. Chronic kidney disease represented 5 billion Medicare dollars in 2006. More than 18,000 kidney transplants were performed in 2006, including deceased and living donors. In a single critical care facility, 67% of patients had acute kidney injury (as defined by the RIFLE criteria; Hoste and Schurgers[1]), with a hazard ratio of 2.7 in predicting mortality.

INDICATIONS FOR NATIVE KIDNEY BIOPSY

Reasons to obtain percutaneous renal biopsy include to establish an exact diagnosis, to plan therapy or decide if therapy is futile, and to determine prognosis.[2] Indications for percutaneous native kidney biopsy vary significantly among clinicians, however. Renal biopsy may also be indicated for patients who possibly have a genetic disease and may benefit from genetic counseling. The overall rate of native percutaneous renal biopsy in number of procedures per million (ppm) population varies from greater than 250 ppm in Australia to less than 75 ppm in the United States.[3]

In adults, nephrotic syndrome (which consists of edema, low serum albumin, proteinuria in excess of 3 g over 24 hours, elevated cholesterol, and hypercoagulability) may be attributable to focal segmental glomeruler sclerosis (FSGS), membranous nephropathy, minimal change disease, membranoproliferative glomerulonephritis, or paraproteinemia. Tissue diagnosis can identify the cause and guide management. Renal biopsy for nephrotic syndrome in adults influenced the management decision in 86% of cases.[4] Percutaneous renal biopsy is usually deferred if there is high clinical suspicion that the nephrotic syndrome is attributable to primary or secondary amyloidosis or diabetes mellitus. If secondary membranous or membranoproliferative glomerulonephritis is found at biopsy, this can point toward a primary autoimmune, neoplastic, or infective process. Most clinicians would agree that a patient should not undergo percutaneous renal biopsy if the results of the biopsy do not change therapeutic management.

As a rule, children with proteinuria are treated empirically with steroids before undergoing renal biopsy, because a significant number of pediatric patients have minimal change disease or steroid-responsive FSGS. Renal biopsies in children younger than the age of 6 years who have nephrotic syndrome may not be necessary, because greater than 90% have minimal change disease. If pediatric patients do not respond to steroid therapy, biopsy may be performed.

Subnephrotic proteinuria is a sign of renal injury in a variety of renal processes, such as obesity, diabetes, obstructive sleep apnea, hypertension, or macrovascular disease. Many clinicians may choose to treat subnephrotic proteinuria

[a] Department of Radiology, University of North Carolina Hospitals, University of North Carolina, Chapel Hill, NC 27599–7510, USA
[b] Department of Nephrology and Hypertension, University of North Carolina Kidney Center, University of North Carolina School of Medicine, 7024 Burnett Womack Building, Chapel Hill, NC 27599, USA
* Corresponding author.
E-mail address: wk_chong@med.unc.edu (W.K. Chong).

Ultrasound Clin 4 (2009) 45–55
doi:10.1016/j.cult.2009.04.001

empirically with angiotensin-converting enzyme inhibitors or angiotensin receptor blockers and defer biopsy if creatinine elevation (glomerular filtration rate depression) occurs along an appropriately predictable course.

Subnephrotic proteinuria can be an indication for biopsy, however, if accompanied by acute kidney injury, an unexplained elevation of creatinine for any length of time, hematuria, or pyuria. Of 151 patients with asymptomatic proteinuria, 10.6% developed renal insufficiency.[5] Asymptomatic hematuria with concurrent proteinuria predicts a poor outcome. In the study by Yamagata and colleagues,[5] the onset of renal insufficiency was observed in 14.9% of 134 patients with asymptomatic hematuria and proteinuria. In patients with urine sediment containing dysmorphic red blood cells, red blood cell casts, or white blood cell casts, most clinicians pursue percutaneous renal biopsy. Patients with subnephrotic proteinuria and positive antinuclear antibody, anti–double-stranded DNA antibody, antineutrophil cytoplasmic antibody, antiglomerular basement membrane (GBM) antibody, or cryoglobulins often undergo renal biopsy. Antineutrophil cytoplasmic antibody and anti-GBM antibodies can present with a rapidly progressive glomerulonephritis that may require emergent biopsy. Other indications for renal biopsy include positive hepatitis serology, rapid plasma reagin, HIV, or parvovirus in the setting of proteinuria. Biopsy is rarely helpful in patients with hematuria alone without proteinuria and with normal creatinine.

Pyuria, with or without proteinuria, can be an indication for biopsy if acute or chronic interstitial nephritis is included in the differential diagnosis. Chronic interstitial nephritis can be attributable to Sjogren's syndrome, sarcoidosis, systemic lupus erythematosus, or drugs, and once the cause is defined, treatment can be pursued or the offending agent can be stopped.

The most common causes of acute renal failure—prerenal disease, acute tubular necrosis, and urinary tract obstruction—can be diagnosed without renal biopsy. The most common cause of creatinine elevation in the hospital is tubular damage from renal injury from nephrotoxins or from hypoxia or hypoperfusion. Often, percutaneous renal biopsy is not indicated in the native kidney if the urine sediment is classic with "muddy-brown casts" or sloughed renal tubular epithelial cells and fatty casts. If the clinician cannot elicit a clear cause for renal injury or does not see a classic pattern in a patient's presentation, however, a renal biopsy may be indicated to rule out a potentially treatable lesion. Richards and colleagues[4] note that renal biopsy altered the management of 22 (71%) of 31 patients with acute renal failure.

Patients with small kidneys or slowly progressive chronic renal failure over a period of years are generally not biopsied, because there is little likelihood of finding a treatable disease (**Fig. 1**).[6] In chronic kidney disease, according to Kobrin[7] and Madaio,[2] clinical suspicion about the cause of renal injury was confirmed by biopsy in only half of patients. In patients who have chronic kidney disease, renal biopsy has a high risk for complications and rarely led to a modification of therapy.[2,7]

INDICATIONS FOR TRANSPLANT KIDNEY BIOPSY

Indications for percutaneous transplant biopsy vary according to time elapsed since the transplant. The kidney may be biopsied at the time of transplantation to obtain a baseline to distinguish preexisting disease from posttransplant pathologic findings.

In the immediate posttransplant period, failure of creatinine to decrease within 1 week (a creatinine plateau) or delayed graft function (requiring dialysis) is an indication for biopsy to evaluate for rejection versus reperfusion injury.

Beyond the immediate postoperative period, elevated creatinine may warrant obtaining a tissue diagnosis. Biopsy is required to diagnose rejection or infection with BK virus, cytomegalovirus, or adenovirus. If treated promptly, rejection can be reversed. The immunosuppressive drugs that are used to prevent rejection, such as calcineurin inhibitors and rapamycin, can themselves lead to graft injury. If morphologic changes likely secondary to medications are seen on biopsy, alteration of medication can save the graft. Biopsy can also identify posttransplant lymphoproliferative disorder. Proteinuria in the setting of preserved glomerular filtration may indicate recurrent FSGS and require biopsy. Recurrent FSGS can be treated with plasmapheresis. Additionally, some centers perform protocol biopsies at set intervals in patients with normal renal function to screen for acute or chronic rejection.

CONTRAINDICATIONS

Absolute contraindications to percutaneous native kidney biopsy were defined in by the Health and Public Policy Committee of the American College of Physicians[8] in 1988, and they are uncontrolled severe hypertension, uncontrollable bleeding diathesis, an uncooperative patient, and a solitary native kidney. Kidneys less than 9 cm in length with increased echogenicity are usually not biopsied, because it is presumed that these kidneys have chronic irreversible disease.

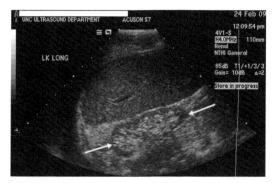

Fig. 1. Small kidney with atrophic cortex indicating end-stage renal disease. Kidneys with cortical thickness of less than 1 cm are usually not biopsied, because the disease process is irreversible.

In other situations, the decision to proceed to biopsy depends on the clinical scenario. A clinician may be more likely to pursue renal biopsy even under less ideal circumstances in the setting of rapidly progressive glomerulonephritis. Conversely, if the patient has numerous contraindications to kidney biopsy and the anticipated renal lesion is potentially less aggressive, biopsy may be deferred. Precautions must be taken when considering a biopsy for a patient on anticoagulation or platelet inhibitors; with prolonged bleeding time; with an elevated international normalized ratio attributable to medical conditions, including disseminated intravascular coagulation and liver failure; anemia with a hemoglobin value less than 8 grams/deciliter, or thrombocytopenia with platelets less than 50×10 9th/L. Aspirin or nonsteroidal anti-inflammatory drugs should be stopped for at least 5 to 7 days before a scheduled elective biopsy, and the patient should remain off of such drugs for at least 1 week after the biopsy. Heparin should be stopped the day before the procedure. The risks of temporarily reversing anticoagulation for the biopsy must be considered for patients on warfarin. Renal failure is associated with platelet dysfunction, anemia, or severe hypertension.[9] Percutaneous renal biopsy should not be pursued in patients with uncontrolled hypertension. Postbiopsy bleeding increased from less than 5% for patients with systolic blood pressure less than 160 mm Hg, to greater than 10% for systolic blood pressure greater than 160 mm Hg.[10] Patients with uremia can be given desmopressin to help normalize bleeding time in the setting of "uremic platelets."

Pregnant or extremely obese patients can be positioned in the seated or lateral decubitus position if the clinician judges the need for the kidney biopsy to justify any increased risk incurred by not being able to lie prone. Most clinicians consider a solitary native kidney, congenital or functional, to be an absolute contraindication to biopsy; therefore, a renal ultrasound scan should precede percutaneous renal biopsy. Biopsy in the presence of hydronephrosis, or passing through a renal cyst or mass, should be avoided whenever possible. Ectopic or polycystic or horseshoe kidneys should not be biopsied. Many clinicians also hesitate to perform biopsy on patients with possible pyelonephritis or perirenal infection or with infection over the skin of the biopsy site.[8]

PROCEDURE
Patient Setup

Informed written consent should be obtained from the patient before the start of the procedure by the person performing the procedure. The risks described should include the risk for bleeding, infection, arteriovenous fistula, and mortality. The platelets, prothrombin time (PT), and partial thromboplastin time (PTT) should all be checked, or recent studies should be available. Any coagulopathy should be appropriately corrected. A blood type and screen should also be available within the blood bank. Anticoagulants, such as aspirin, warfarin, or enoxaparin, should have been stopped at least 1 week before the biopsy. Subcutaneous enoxaparin should be held for a minimum of 12 hours before the procedure. Vital signs should be monitored throughout the procedure. Large-bore intravenous access should be in place. At the authors' institution, the procedure is performed under conscious sedation and a combination of fentanyl and midazolam is used. In neonates and small children, the procedure is performed under general anesthesia.

Prebiopsy Scan

During the prescan, both kidneys are evaluated for size, cortical thickness, and echogenicity,

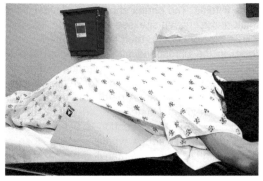

Fig. 2. Prone native kidney biopsy position. A posterior approach is used for native kidneys. The wedge is placed under the abdomen to eliminate the lumbar lordosis.

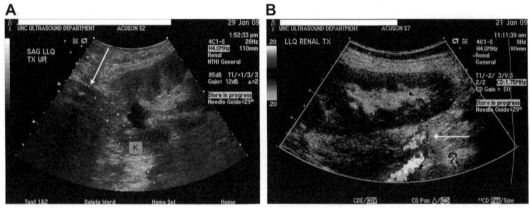

Fig. 3. Pitfalls. (*A*) Longitudinal image of transplant kidney with electronic marker lines shows that gas-filled bowel (linear echogenicity with posterior shadowing, *arrow*) lies in the way of the trajectory of the needle to the cortex (K). (*B*) Iliac vessels (*arrow*) lie in the needle trajectory deep to the lower pole of the transplant kidney.

hydronephrosis, or perinephric fluid collections. The kidney is evaluated for hydronephrosis, cysts, stones, or masses. Color Doppler flow is used to identify blood vessels within the kidney and along the potential biopsy route. Biopsies should be obtained as close to the periphery of the kidney as possible, where the blood vessels are smallest, to minimize bleeding. This also maximizes the amount of cortex in the specimen. For native kidneys, the lower pole is the optimal site (the upper pole is more difficult to reach because of overlying ribs). The left kidney is traditionally preferred to avoid transgressing the liver; however, either kidney can be biopsied. The renal hilum, which contains the main renal artery, vein, and their major branches and collecting system, should be avoided. The optimal route to the target is identified, and the distance from the skin is measured during the prescan. The route chosen should be the shortest one possible without passing through bowel, ribs, bone, or large vessels. The targeted area of the kidney should not contain cysts, masses, calculi, or arteriovenous fistulae. The cortex should be at least 1 cm thick at the chosen site (see **Fig. 1**).

The biopsy is performed in a dedicated biopsy room in the ultrasound suite. This room should be large enough to contain monitoring and resuscitation equipment in addition to sterile supplies needed for the biopsy. A pathology technician is present on-site to determine adequacy of the specimen. Conscious sedation is used with fentanyl and midazolam. A typical starting dose of midazolam is 1 mg; for fentanyl, a typical starting dose is 150 µg. An appropriate level of analgesia requires that the patient be arousable and able to follow commands. Vital signs are monitored by a nurse throughout the procedure. The patient is

positioned in the prone position for a native kidney target and in the supine position for a transplant kidney. Rolled towels or a wedge is placed under the abdomen to eliminate the lumbar lordosis (**Fig. 2**). At the authors' institution, the biopsy is normally performed by nephrologists with real-time sonographic guidance from trained sonographers. Although the procedure can be performed freehand, the authors prefer to use a built-in guide to improve accuracy.

If overlying bowel gas (**Fig. 3**), vessels, or hydronephrosis (**Fig. 4**) is identified during the prescan, an alternative route should be found that avoids transgressing these structures. **Fig. 4** demonstrates a planned renal biopsy that was postponed secondary to severe hydronephrosis.

The path of the needle is indicated on the video display by a dotted line or two parallel dotted lines. The dots are spaced 1 cm apart. The angle of the dotted lines can be adjusted to the angle chosen on the guide. The biopsy guide on the authors' equipment allows a choice between two angles: 18 and 32 (**Fig. 5**). Once the appropriate angle

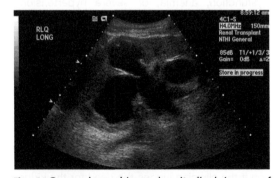

Fig. 4. Gray-scale prebiopsy longitudinal image of a renal transplant demonstrating severe hydronephrosis, a contraindication to biopsy.

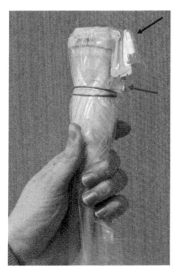

Fig. 5. Biopsy guide. The guide consists of outer and inner components. The latter is attached to the transducer by means of a coupler. The metal knob on the inner component (*red arrow*) allows a choice of two approach angles by slotting in one of the two notches on the coupler. A sterile sheath is placed over the coupled transducer. The outer component is a sterile disposable insert (*arrow*) that mates with the inner component over the sterile sheath. When the inner and outer components are joined, a tunnel is created through which the biopsy needle is passed.

has been determined, the transducer and guide are draped with a sterile cover. A sterile disposable insert is attached to the covered guide. Inserts can accommodate needles of different sizes; for core

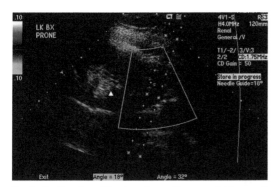

Fig. 6. Optimal positioning for native renal biopsy. A longitudinal image of the left kidney is obtained with the patient in the prone position lying over a wedge as in **Fig. 2**. There is no hydronephrosis. The needle passes between the two parallel dotted electronic marker lines. The dots are at 1-cm intervals. The needle tract is aimed at the lower pole renal parenchyma, avoiding the echogenic renal sinus (*arrowhead*). Color Doppler imaging shows no major vessels, bowel, or other vital structures along the projected needle path superficial to or beyond the kidney.

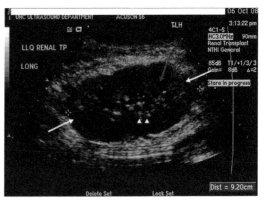

Fig. 7. Longitudinal image of a renal transplant. The glomeruli, located in the cortex, are the site of most cases of renal parenchymal disease. The optimal place for biopsy is the upper or lower pole cortex (*white arrows*), avoiding the echogenic renal sinus, where the main renal artery, vein, and collecting system are located (*arrowhead*). This maximizes the number of glomeruli and reduces bleeding complications. The medulla (*red arrow*) is a triangular hypoechoic structure situated between the cortex and the echogenic renal sinus. In transplants, some medullary tissue is required for diagnosis when FSGS is suspected.

biopsies, an insert one size larger than the biopsy needle is used, allowing the outer sheath of the biopsy gun to slide freely when it is fired (see **Fig. 5**). As a rule, the electronic biopsy cursors that mark the tract of the needle should pass through the hypoechoic renal parenchyma, avoiding the renal sinus fat (**Fig. 6**). The biopsy tract should not pass through major vessels, such as the iliac artery or aorta beyond the kidney, in case the operator overshoots (see **Fig. 3**). A similar

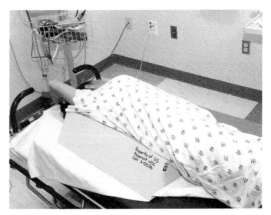

Fig. 8. Right anterior oblique position for biopsy of a right lower quadrant renal transplant. The right anterior oblique position facilitates a lateral approach, which is useful for avoiding overlying bowel.

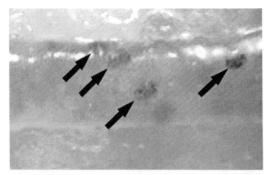

Fig. 9. Renal biopsy specimen with the flush of glomeruli (*arrows*). (*Courtesy of* Dr. J.C. Jennette, MD, Chapel Hill, NC.)

approach should be taken for transplant kidneys to minimize risk to the iliac vessels.

Most transplant kidneys are located in the right or left lower quadrant in an extraperitoneal location (**Fig. 7**). Overlying bowel can be a significant problem. The upper or lower pole can be used. For transplant kidneys, the patient is placed in the supine or left lateral decubitus position if the kidney is in the right lower quadrant and in the right lateral decubitus if the kidney is in the left lower quadrant (**Fig. 8**). The decubitus positions are used if there is overlying bowel gas in the supine position.

The native kidney moves inferiorly with inspiration. The degree of respiratory excursion varies with individual patients but can be considerable. Biopsies of native kidneys are performed in suspended respiration. Practice breath-holds should be performed with the patient during the prebiopsy scan. Transplant kidneys usually do not move during respiration, and suspended respiration is not necessary.

The skin site is prepared in a sterile manner and is then appropriately draped. The selection of biopsy needles is a matter of operator preference. Typically 14- to 16-gauge needles are used. The length of the needle is determined by the distance of the target from the skin. Spring-loaded needles are preferred because they can be operated with one hand, whereas disposable non-spring fired needles type needles require both hands. Spring-loaded needles have throws of between 2 and 3 cm, although some needles have adjustable throws. The larger gauge needles are generally associated with increased risk for bleeding-associated complications but are also associated with more glomeruli per sample, requiring fewer passes to achieve adequacy.[11] Spring-loaded needles are preferred because they can be operated one-handed, whereas the older disposable non-spring fired needles/Vim-Silverman type needles require both hands.

BIOPSY

After the biopsy site has been appropriately prepared, local anesthetic (2% lidocaine) is administered superficially at the skin site and then along the intended biopsy tract through the soft tissues, especially if the biopsy course must pass through muscle. If the administration of lidocaine is painful to the patient, a 4:1 mixture of lidocaine/sodium bicarbonate can be used to minimize the discomfort. A small nick at the intended skin entrance site should be made to allow ready passage of the biopsy needle.

The biopsy needle is placed into the guide, and the needle tip is inserted into the skin incision. The transducer is moved down the needle and placed on the skin. At this point, final adjustments in direction can be made. The needle is then advanced

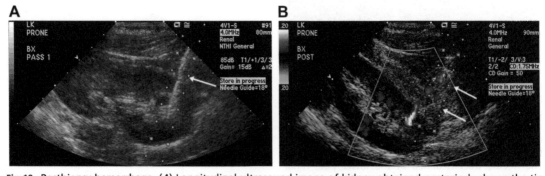

Fig. 10. Postbiopsy hemorrhage. (*A*) Longitudinal ultrasound image of kidney obtained posteriorly shows the tip of the biopsy needle between biopsy markers penetrating the echogenic sinus of the kidney. This increases the risk for bleeding. (*B*) Postbiopsy image demonstrates anterior displacement of the lower pole of the kidney, which now lies at a greater distance from the skin because of perinephric hematoma (*white arrows*). Color Doppler component of the image demonstrates an active bleed (*red arrow*) from the biopsy site.

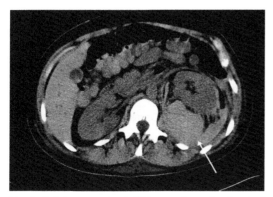

Fig. 11. Axial noncontrast CT image from the level of the kidneys 1 day after biopsy. A large hyperdense hematoma lies posterior to the left kidney. The kidney is displaced anteriorly.

toward the kidney under real-time sonographic guidance. The sonographer should aim to keep the needle tip in view at all times. If the tip cannot be clearly seen, a gentle up and down motion of the needle or rocking of the transducer can aid visualization. Visualization of the needle can be difficult or impossible in obese patients because of the echogenicity of the abdominal wall fat. In that situation, the operator has to estimate the depth of the needle by tissue motion. Respiration should be suspended before the tip of the needle enters the kidney. The firing mechanism is activated when the tip of the needle is at or just past the renal capsule. The needle travels the length of the throw when fired; thus, care should be taken that there are no vital structures in the path of the needle. An image or video clip of the needle position during biopsy should be recorded and saved. After the needle is withdrawn, the sonographer scans the needle tract with Doppler imaging to look for evidence of bleeding, free fluid, or hematoma. Hematoma appears as a mixed-echogenicity solid mass overlying the biopsy site. A hematoma may be difficult to see because it is isoechoic with the perinephric tissue, but a useful indicator of hematoma size is a postbiopsy increase in the skin-to-lesion distance compared with the prebiopsy scan. Only if bleeding is extremely active does blood appear transsonic. As each sample is acquired, it is handed to the pathology technician for evaluation under light microscopy. If there is no evidence of complications, repeat passes may be taken until adequate diagnostic material has been obtained.

SPECIMEN ADEQUACY

For some diseases, such as membranous glomerulonephritis or Alport syndrome, the diagnosis can be made with a single glomerulus. In most cases, however, more glomeruli are needed and a larger volume of renal tissue is required to make a reliable diagnosis.[2] Crescentic glomerulonephritis requires more glomeruli to make the diagnosis. Incorrect classification could occur in diseases in which the percentage of affected glomeruli categorizes patients into separate groups, as is the case in lupus erythematosus. In native kidney biopsy, statistical analysis has shown that more than 20 glomeruli for light microscopy are sufficient to exclude sampling error, even in cases with a low frequency of glomerular lesions.[12] Therefore, it is crucial that the biopsy cores are checked to determine specimen adequacy during the procedure and further passes can then be obtained if necessary.[13] With a laboratory microscope on low power (×5), kidney tissue can be discriminated from fat or muscle and it is possible to count the number of glomeruli within a biopsy core and estimate the proportion of cortex contained in the sample (**Fig. 9**). A transplant biopsy sample is considered adequate when a specimen

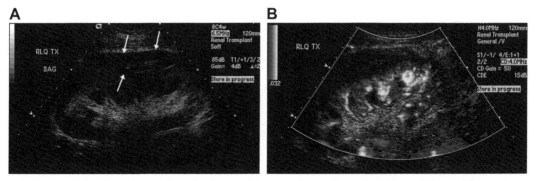

Fig. 12. Gray-scale (*top*) and power Doppler (*bottom*) images of a posttransplant biopsy kidney with an intracapsular hematoma recognizable by its lenticular shape (*arrow*). Pressure from the hematoma can lead to a Page kidney. The power Doppler signal only extends to the cortical edge of the kidney but not into the subcapsular hematoma.

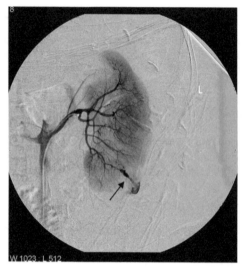

Fig. 13. Angiogram shows contrast extravasation from an arteriole in the lower pole of the kidney (*arrow*) secondary to biopsy.

contains 10 or more glomeruli and two arteries.[14] A minimal sample is 7 glomeruli and one artery. There should be two cores of tissues containing cortex or two separate areas of cortex in the same core.[15] Medulla is needed in the biopsy sample when evaluating transplant kidneys or when evaluating for FSGS (typically in proteinuric patients). Electron microscopy is performed on biopsy samples, except for those from kidneys within a year of transplantation, unless FSGS is the primary cause of renal failure.

POSTBIOPSY MONITORING

At the authors' institution, renal biopsies are performed as outpatient procedures. Once the biopsy is completed, the patient is transferred to the nursing hold area, where vitals signs are monitored on a standardized schedule. The patient remains supine for 6 hours after biopsy and should have vital signs closely monitored, with blood pressures to be maintained lower than 140/90. Short-acting beta-blockers may be used to lower the blood pressure. A repeat renal ultrasound scan is obtained to follow hematoma size and reassess for active bleeding. During this time, the urine is racked to evaluate for clots or gross hematuria and to follow hematuria clearance. Hemoglobin should be reassessed 6 hours after biopsy to ensure that the patient has not had bleeding requiring transfusion. If the 4-hour ultrasound scan demonstrates no complications, the patient is discharged. If there is evidence of active

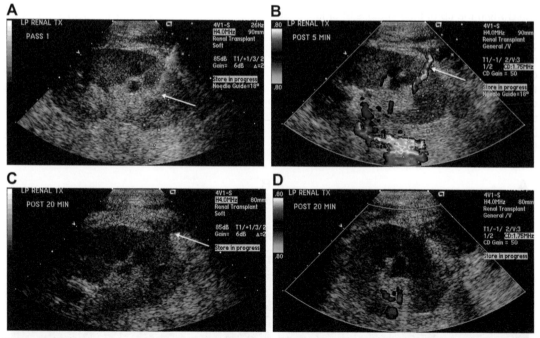

Fig. 14. Multiple gray-scale and Doppler ultrasound images of a native kidney. (*A*) Initial image demonstrates the biopsy needle penetrating the echogenic renal sinus (hyperechoic area, *arrow*) in the transplant kidney. (*B*) Subsequent color Doppler images at 5 minutes after biopsy demonstrate an active bleed. Compression was then applied to the transplant kidney. At 20 minutes after biopsy, gray-scale (*C*) and Doppler (*D*) images demonstrate cessation of bleeding. A small perinephric hematoma (*arrow*) is seen.

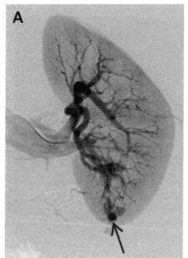

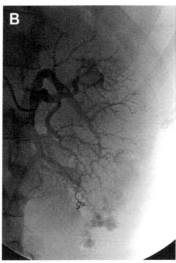

Fig. 15. False aneurysm. (*A*) Rounded density (*arrow*) represents the false aneurysm in the lower pole of the kidney. (*B*) Aneurysm is ablated after selective embolization of its feeding artery. An embolization coil is seen at the lower pole.

bleeding, such as a growing hematoma or hematuria, the patient is admitted overnight for monitoring.

The most common complication from renal biopsy is a clinically insignificant perinephric hematoma that is only apparent on ultrasound.[16] This may be visualized on postbiopsy scans as a heterogenous mass on the surface of the kidney at the biopsy site. Larger hematomas may cause a drop in hematocrit or pain and may lead to urinary tract obstruction. Sonographically, they may appear as an increase in the distance between the kidney and skin surface (**Figs. 10** and **11**). Distortion of the renal contour may indicate a subcapsular hematoma.[17] Pressure caused by a subcapsular hematoma within the confined subcapsular space can result in hypertension and renal failure (**Fig. 12**).

Active hemorrhage (see **Fig. 10; Fig. 13**) may usually be identified on the immediate postbiopsy

or the follow-up postbiopsy ultrasound scan using color Doppler imaging. Simple compression may be sufficient to stop active bleeding in transplant kidneys. **Fig. 14** demonstrates the cessation of active bleeding by compression in a transplant kidney. Bleeding from native kidneys cannot usually be mitigated by compression. Risk factors for bleeding include hypertension, renal insufficiency, and anemia.[9,16,18,19] Bleeding can be minimized by ensuring that patients have a normal PTT, PT, platelet count, and bleeding time. Avoiding the renal sinus fat and the large vessels it contains also reduces the risk for bleeding (see **Figs. 10** and **14**). In one retrospective study of 645 renal biopsies, postbiopsy bleeding occurred in 2% and 12% of patients with a serum creatinine concentration lower than or greater than 2 mg/dL, respectively.[9] Bleeding severe enough to cause hypotension occurs in 1% to 2% of biopsies, and bleeding severe enough to require transfusion occurs in up to 6% of biopsies. Surgery is required to control bleeding in 0.1% to 0.4% of biopsies, with a nephrectomy rate of 0.3%. The quoted risk for mortality is 0.02% to 0.1%.[2,9,18,20,21] A decrease in hemoglobin level of 1 g/dL or more is a complication in approximately 50% of biopsies. In most cases, active bleeding after biopsy ceases spontaneously. If immediate or postbiopsy imaging demonstrates a hemorrhage that cannot be controlled with manual compression or other noninvasive techniques, immediate embolization or surgery may be required.

Another potential complication from biopsy is the creation of an arteriovenous fistula or pseudoaneurysm. The vascularity of the kidney and invasive nature of the biopsy naturally lend themselves to the formation of arteriovenous shunts. If

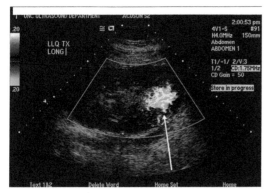

Fig. 16. Postbiopsy false aneurysm, shown as an area of heterogenous Doppler signal attributable to turbulence in the lower pole of the kidney.

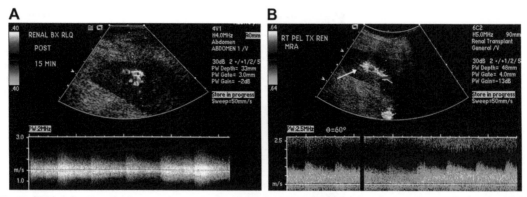

Fig. 17. (*Top*) Color Doppler images demonstrate an arteriovenous fistula with turbulent flow in the region of the fistula. (*Bottom*) Color and spectral Doppler images of the same kidney covering the area of the main renal artery. The renal artery supplying the arteriovenous fistula (*arrow*) demonstrates low-resistance flow, consistent with significant hemodynamic shunting through the arteriovenous fistula.

a biopsy needle penetrates a sufficiently large arteriole, a contained leak or pseudoaneurysm can form (**Fig. 15**). Arteriovenous fistulae are created when the needle penetrates an artery and a venule, creating a communication between them. Arteriovenous fistulae and pseudoaneurysms are visible on color Doppler imaging as a splash of mosaic color within the kidney along the biopsy tract (**Fig. 16**). Spectral Doppler imaging demonstrates characteristic turbulent high-velocity low-resistance flow with spectral broadening. Small arteriovenous fistulas are usually asymptomatic and of no clinical consequence. Care, however, should be taken to avoid biopsying areas with arteriovenous fistulas to prevent enlargement. Large arteriovenous fistulas may result in renal failure, high-output cardiac

failure, or thromboembolic phenomenon. Once an arteriovenous fistula is identified, the interventionalist may provide relief using coil embolization. **Figs. 17** and **18** demonstrate a large postbiopsy arteriovenous fistula in a transplant kidney.

Transient microscopic hematuria occurs in almost all patients. Postbiopsy CT scan evidence of an intrarenal or perinephric hematoma occurs in 60% to 80% of patients. Transient gross hematuria is noted in 3% to 12%. Gross blood in the urine may also cause blood clots to form; these clots may cause subsequent obstruction of the ureters and subsequent hydronephrosis. This may be identified by a combination of decreased urine output and observation of hydronephrosis on subsequent ultrasound imaging.

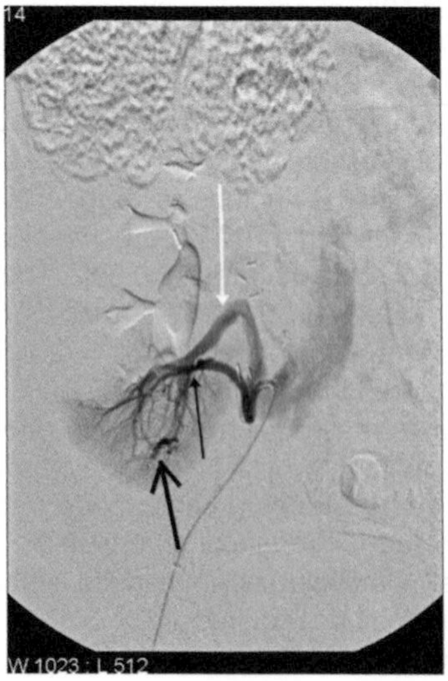

RADIOLOGIC MANAGEMENT OF COMPLICATIONS

Coil embolization is the preferred method for controlling postbiopsy bleeds that cannot be managed medically.[22] A direct angiogram of the renal artery is performed to identify the bleeding site, followed by selective canalization of the bleeding vessel. Once in position, embolization coils may be delivered to the bleeding vessel at a location proximal to the bleed. **Fig. 15** demonstrates angiographic evidence of a false aneurysm and subsequent successful coil embolization. Permanent embolization techniques are needed to prevent rebleeding secondary to the constant arterial pressure. Postembolization angiography should confirm the cessation of bleeding. Arteriovenous fistulas may be treated in a similar manner.[23,24]

SUMMARY

Sonography is an excellent modality for guidance of renal biopsy. Ultrasound can detect potential pitfalls, direct proper placement of the needle,

Fig. 18. Corresponding angiogram to **Fig. 13**. The right lower pole renal artery has been selectively catheterized. An arteriovenous fistula (*black arrow*) is shown with premature filling of the renal vein (*white arrow*).

and identify complications. Interventional radiology or surgical support should be available in the event of complications.

REFERENCES

1. Hoste EAJ, Schurgers M. Epidemiology of acute kidney injury: how big is the problem? Crit Care Med 2008;36(Suppl 4):S146–51.
2. Madaio MP. Renal biopsy. Kidney Int 1990;38(3): 529–43.
3. Briganti EM, Dowling J, Finlay M, et al. The incidence of biopsy-proven glomerulonephritis in Australia. Nephrol Dial Transplant 2001;16(7):1364–7.
4. Richards NT, Darby S, Howie AJ, et al. Knowledge of renal histology alters patient management in over 40% of cases. Nephrol Dial Transplant 1994;9(9): 1255–9.
5. Yamagata K, Yamagata Y, Kobayashi M, et al. A long-term follow-up study of asymptomatic hematuria and/or proteinuria in adults. Clin Nephrol 1996;45(5):281–8.
6. Tomson CRV. Indications for renal biopsy in chronic kidney disease. Clin Med 2003;3(6):513–7.
7. Kobrin S, Madaio MP. Renal biopsy. In: The principles and practice of nephrology. St. Louis (MO): Mosby; 1996. p. 65–71.
8. Health and Public Policy Committee, American College of Physicians. Clinical competence in percutaneous renal biopsy. Ann Intern Med 1988; 108(2):301–3.
9. Shidham GB, Siddiqi N, Beres JA, et al. Clinical risk factors associated with bleeding after native kidney biopsy. Nephrology (Carlton) 2005;10(3):305–10.
10. Stiles KP, Hill C, LeBrun CJ, et al. The impact of bleeding times on major complication rates after percutaneous real-time ultrasound-guided renal biopsies. J Nephrol 2001;14(4):275–9.
11. Doyle AJ, Gregory MC, Terreros DA. Percutaneous native renal biopsy: comparison of a 1.2-mm spring-driven system with a traditional 2-mm hand-driven system. Am J Kidney Dis 1994;23(4): 498–503.
12. Corwin HL, Schwartz MM, Lewis EJ. The importance of sample size in the interpretation of the renal biopsy. Am J Nephrol 1988;8(2):85–9.
13. Pirani CL, Croker B. Handling and processing of renal biopsy and nephrectomy specimens. In: Tisher CC, Brenner BM, editors. Renal pathology, vol. 2. 2nd edition. Philadelphia: J.B. Lippincott Co.; 1994. p. 1683–94.
14. Racusen LC, Solez K, Colvin RB, et al. The Banff 97 working classification of renal allograft pathology. Kidney Int 1999;55(2):713–23.
15. Amann K, Haas CS. What you should know about the work-up of a renal biopsy. Nephrol Dial Transplant 2006;21(5):1157–61.
16. Eiro M, Katoh T, Watanabe T. Risk factors for bleeding complications in percutaneous renal biopsy. Clin Exp Nephrol 2005;9(1):40–5.
17. Marshall WH, Castellino RA. Hypertension produced by constricting capsular renal lesions. ("Page" kidney). Radiology 1971;101(3):561–5.
18. Korbet SM. Percutaneous renal biopsy. Semin Nephrol 2002;22(3):254–67.
19. Whittier WL, Korbet SM. Timing of complications in percutaneous renal biopsy. J Am Soc Nephrol 2004;15(1):142–7.
20. Mendelssohn DC, Cole EH. Outcomes of percutaneous kidney biopsy, including those of solitary native kidneys. Am J Kidney Dis 1995;26(4):580–5.
21. Parrish AE. Complications of percutaneous renal biopsy: a review of 37 years' experience. Clin Nephrol 1992;38(3):135–41.
22. Perini S, Gordon RL, LaBerge JM, et al. Transcatheter embolization of biopsy-related vascular injury in the transplant kidney: immediate and long-term outcome. J Vasc Interv Radiol 1998;9(6):1011–9.
23. Hübsch P, Schurawitzki H, Traindl O, et al. Renal allograft arteriovenous fistula due to needle biopsy with late onset of symptoms—diagnosis and treatment. Nephron 1991;59(3):482–5.
24. Loffroy R, Guiu B, Lambert A, et al. Management of post-biopsy renal allograft arteriovenous fistulas with selective arterial embolization: immediate and long-term outcomes. Clin Radiol 2008;63(6): 657–65.

Ultrasound-Guided Radiofrequency Ablation Within the Abdomen

John P. McGahan, MD*, Wayne Monsky, MD, PhD

KEYWORDS

- Radiofrequency ablation • Liver • Kidney
- Percutaneous ethanol ablation • Interventional
- Ultrasound interventional • CT

Many patients with either hepatic or renal malignancies are not candidates for potential curative surgery. As such, investigators have searched for safe alternative methods of treatment of these lesions to help control and cure disease and avoid the potential morbidity associated with surgery. Image guidance is needed for percutaneous needle placement using these modalities. Ultrasound or CT or a combination of the two modalities can be used for needle placement and to guide therapy.

Before the advent of CT fluoroscopy, only sonography and radiographic fluoroscopy could be used for real-time needle placement into the abdomen. In our facility, if a lesion is identified by sonography and there is a safe approach, ultrasound is the imaging modality of choice to guide needle placement and monitor therapy for percutaneous tissue ablation. Ultrasound is ideal for several reasons. It is much more widely available worldwide and is used more frequently to guide percutaneous interventional procedures compared with CT. In most countries and in many hospitals, CT time is at a premium. Alternatively, ultrasound is fairly cost-effective and portable and can be transported to a patient's bedside or to any portion of the hospital for guidance of interventional procedures. Sonography, with its real-time capabilities, can guide precise needle placement into small target lesions and is helpful for monitoring therapeutic applications such as radiofrequency ablation (RFA). This article focuses on the use of ultrasound in guidance of percutaneous tissue ablation within the abdomen. The main focus of this article is use of ultrasound-guided RFA within the liver and the kidney, whether alone or in combination with other techniques.

Percutaneous tissue ablation has followed an interesting path. Although many of the technical applications and innovations for tissue ablation have occurred only recently, there has been a long history of use of interstitial therapy either performed at surgery or performed percutaneously. For instance, as early as 1979, Tabuse[1] described a new operative procedure of hepatic surgery to allow surgeons to transect liver parenchyma and coagulate the cut surface simultaneously using microwave hyperthermia. Microwave hyperthermia was later described in the early 1990s, guided by ultrasound to perform percutaneous coagulation therapy for small hepatocellular carcinomas (HCCs).[2] Hashimoto described the use of Nd:YAG laser for malignant tumors of the liver in 1985, which was guided by sonography.[3] Cryotherapy of the liver was described in the early 1990s by Onik as a method of treatment of liver cancer.[4] This technique was performed at the time of open surgery, often with sonographic guidance. More recently, however, smaller probes have been developed for performance of percutaneous cryotherapy. Thus percutaneous cryotherapy has been performed in the liver and the kidney.

Worldwide, probably two different techniques have been used more commonly than any other

Department of Radiology, University of California, Davis Medical Center, 4860 Y Street, Suite 3100, Sacramento, CA, 95817, USA
* Corresponding author.
E-mail address: john.mcgahan@ucdmc.ucdavis.edu (J.P. McGahan).

Ultrasound Clin 4 (2009) 57–71
doi:10.1016/j.cult.2009.03.002

to treat either liver or renal malignancies: percutaneous ethanol injection (PEI) and RFA. Livraghi in Italy described the use of percutaneous alcohol injection to treat small HCCs in 1988.[5] Out of Asia, Shiina in 1990 also described the use of ethanol injection for therapy for HCC.[6] Ethanol ablation has several advantages and disadvantages over other technologies. In countries where HCC is more frequent, limited resources may not allow purchase of high-end equipment for treatment such as cryotherapy. Ethanol, as absolute alcohol, is readily available and inexpensive, however. It has been widely used worldwide. Some of the disadvantages of ethanol are that it may require multiple treatments for complete ablation and it is used mainly—but not exclusively—for small hepatomas (< 3 cm). It is not useful for other hepatic malignancies, such as colorectal metastases because these metastases are so "firm" that the alcohol cannot disperse within the lesion.

Another technology that has become fairly popular on a global basis is radiofrequency electrocautery, which was described by McGahan in 1990.[7] McGahan's article described use of focal application of radiofrequency energy in the animal liver using sonographic guidance and monopolar electrocautery with an 18- to 20-gauge needle. The distal tip of the needle was uninsulated, and with application of current an echogenic lesion was observed by ultrasound. Pathologically, the echogenic lesion corresponded to an area of coagulation necrosis. The authors believed that this percutaneous technique had great potential because (1) the lesion was well controlled, (2) the technique allowed for potential re-treatment, (3) there seemed to be the potential for few complications, (4) it could be performed without hospitalization, and (5) the technique could be combined with other therapeutic methods.

Initial research with RFA concentrated on the use of a single monopolar probe for tissue ablation. The radiofrequency probes or needles were insulated except for the distal tip, which allowed for current flow and coagulation necrosis of surrounding tissues. It was soon discovered, however, that the lesions were limited to diameters of 1 to 1.5 cm. With time, there has been refinement of RF technology, with different authors demonstrating novel methods to create larger areas of tissue necrosis. For example, Goldberg and colleagues[8] demonstrated that increased tissue destruction could be performed using multiple probes. Lorentzen[9] demonstrated that using a "cooled" needle electrode with RFA did increase volume of tissue coagulation. Gili and colleagues[10] described the use of a multi-tine probe (Leveen needle) in radiofrequency needles

to increase the volume of tissue coagulation. In this article, methods of RFA and the use of different techniques and problematic areas are discussed in more detail.

MATERIALS AND PROTOCOLS: PERCUTANEOUS ABLATION

The steps taken when deciding to perform RFA or any other percutaneous ablation technique include the following:

   The lesion is identified with CT or MRI or both. It is important to note the relation of the mass to adjacent structures, such as the diaphragm, gallbladder, and adjacent bowel, for liver lesions or the ureter or adjacent bowel for kidney lesions.

   The size of the lesion should be noted carefully. For instance, most tumors smaller than 3 to 4 cm generally are amenable to treatment with RFA or other ablative techniques. Treatment with complete ablation is less successful with larger tumors. In these situations, either surgery or combined techniques might be considered.

   The physician also should assess whether certain factors may preclude RFA, such as intractable, prolonged bleeding times or lack of an appropriate path for needle placement.

   It must be decided if the lesion to be ablated is benign or malignant (**Figs. 1** and **2**). For instance, in patients with new liver lesions and a history of cancer at another site, fine needle aspiration biopsy is usually performed before RFA. For primary lesions in the liver, needle biopsy may or may not be performed. Generally if there is a new enhancing, well-encapsulated mass that has typical CT features of hepatoma and an elevation of alpha fetoprotein, then probably no biopsy is necessary. Biopsy may be performed to determine if the mass is a well-differentiated or poorly differentiated HCC. Alternatively, renal lesion biopsy, which is often performed before treatment, has shown that these solid masses may be benign tumors such as oncocytomas or non–fat-containing angiomyolipomas.

   The physician must decide which imaging modality should be used for needle placement: ultrasound, CT, or a combination of the two. Our preference is to use a combination of ultrasound and CT. It may be

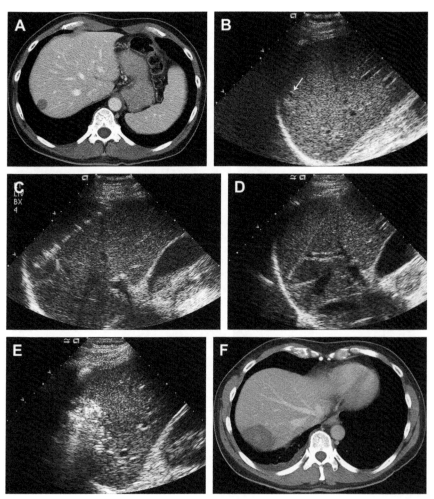

Fig. 1. A 50-year-old patient with isolated liver metastases for RFA and liver biopsy. (*A*) CT scan demonstrates isolated lesion, posterior aspect of right lobe of the liver, in which a biopsy was requested before RFA. (*B*) Ultrasound demonstrates the fairly well-encapsulated echogenic mass noted at the dome of the diaphragm (*arrow*). (*C*) Using a coaxial technique, fine-needle aspiration biopsy revealed metastatic melanoma. (*D*) Two weeks after completing biopsy, RF needle is positioned within the lesion. (*E*) After RFA, large echogenic response is noted. (*F*) Follow-up enhanced CT scan demonstrates the small high-density treated lesion noted centrally within the large low-density ablation zone. Also note small pleural effusion.

decided before procedure which needle is to be used. For instance, if there is a 3-cm lesion, a needle with electrodes that expand to 4 or 5 cm may be used to ensure adequate tumor treatment and a margin of normal liver, which is ablated surrounding the tumor. Likewise, a single, clustered, or multiple cooled tip needle may be used, depending on the size of the lesion.

Before performing the procedure, ultrasound is used to view the intended needle path (**Fig. 3**). This procedure is helpful to visualize potential vessels that may be in the path so they may be avoided during RF needle placement.

Once ultrasound is decided for needle placement, the RF needle is placed into the target lesion under real-time control. If a combination technique such as ethanol ablation plus RFA is to be performed, we usually place the RF needle within the lesion and then place the needle for ethanol ablation (**Fig. 4**). We perform ethanol ablation first, followed by RFA, because we often have found that the echogenic response after ethanol ablation does not readily disappear as quickly as the echogenic response after RFA.

After the RF needle is placed into the lesion, the position of the needle tip may be

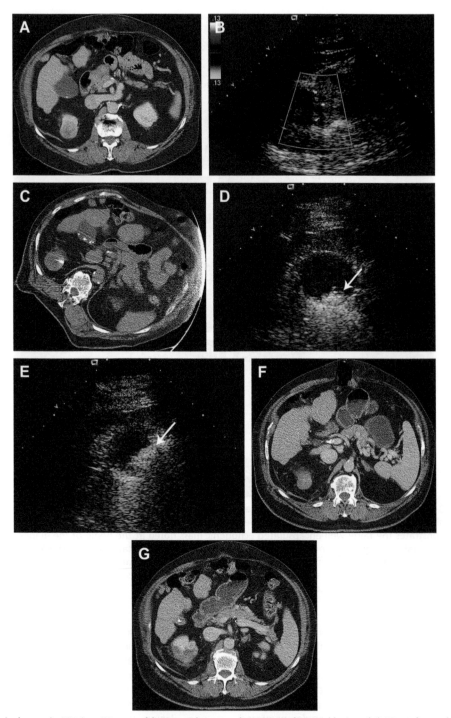

Fig. 2. Typical steps in RFA in a 71-year-old man with new enhancing right renal lesion. (*A*) CT performed for other reasons identified approximately 3-cm enhancing mass, upper pole of the right kidney. Subsequently this mass was biopsied and determined to be renal cell carcinoma. Patient was referred for RFA. (*B*) Ultrasound image is obtained to demonstrate vascularity of the mass and any vessels that should be avoided during needle puncture. (*C*) After RF needle is placed, position is rechecked with CT scan. (*D*) Needle has been positioned with ultrasound, and after initial start of RFA, echogenic response is observed toward the needle tip (*arrow*). (*E*) With increasing treatment there is increasing echogenicity (*arrow*). The needle is then repositioned to regions that may not have been treated completely. This may be done by performing enhanced CT and/or contrast-enhanced ultrasound (if outside the United States). (*F, G*) Follow-up CT scan demonstrates defect in posterior parenchyma of the right kidney and avascular region in location of the right renal cell carcinoma.

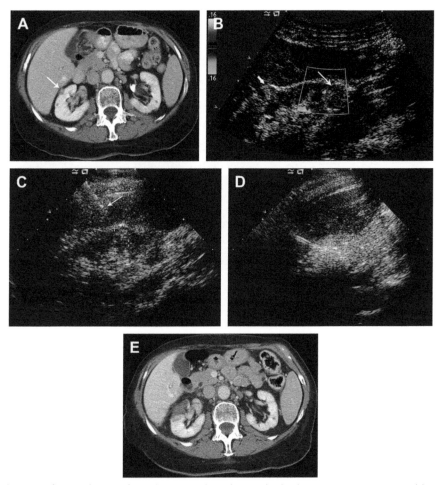

Fig. 3. Renal RFA performed by transhepatic approach and using hydrodissection in an 82-year-old woman with two solid masses in the right kidney. (*A*) CT scan of the smaller lesion identified anterior aspect midpole right kidney (*arrow*). (*B*) Longitudinal ultrasound examination demonstrates well-encapsulated mid-pole lesion (*short arrow*) and lower pole lesion with color flow (*long arrow*). (*C*) RFA needle being placed transhepatically (*arrow*) into mid-pole lesion. (*D*) Echogenic response after ablation of mid-pole lesion. (*E*) Follow-up CT of lesion 1 demonstrates nonenhancement of this area of the kidney.

checked with CT to ensure that it is not in close proximity to vital organs, such as the gallbladder, bowel, or ureter. If the needle is close to structures such as the bowel, diaphragm, or gallbladder, modification of this technique is available, including combination with ethanol injection or use of artificial ascites (**Figs. 5, 6, 7,** and **8**).

After ensuring proper needle placement, RFA may be performed. The ultrasound is useful for monitoring the echogenic response with ablation.

After RFA has been performed, the needle is removed under ultrasound guidance. We usually perform cauterization of the needle track during removal of the needle. Needle removal should be followed closely by ultrasound so as not to cause inadvertent injury to the skin or subcutaneous tissue-track cauterization.

After removal of the needle, the site is checked by ultrasound to ensure that no significant complication is present, such as an arterial or venous fistula from the liver through the liver capsule (see **Fig. 7**).

PROCEDURE NOTES

After completion of the therapy and confirmation of adequate distribution of destructive agent, the patient is monitored for site-specific and systemic complications. We often administer broad-spectrum antibiotics for several days. Combination

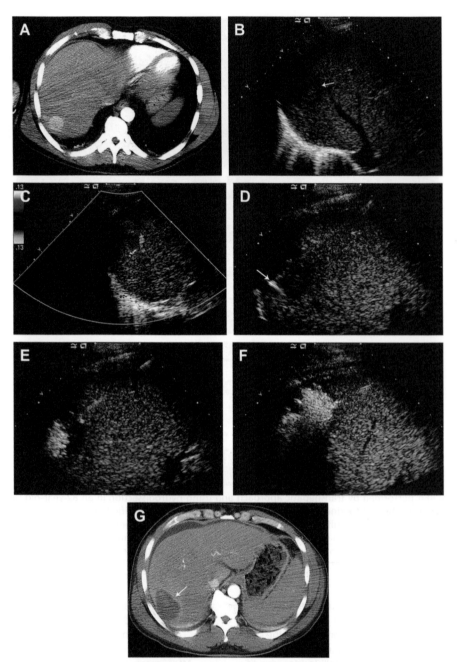

Fig. 4. A 50-year-old man with HCC in segment 7 of the liver for ethanol and RFA ablation. (*A*) Arterial phase CT scan demonstrates enhancing mass in the posterior aspect right lobe of the liver. (*B*) Ultrasound image demonstrates well-encapsulated hypoechoic mass (*arrow*) in the posterior right lobe of the liver. (*C*) Ultrasound image with color demonstrates arterial flow at the periphery of the lesion and hepatic vein adjacent to the lesion demonstrated in blue. (*D*) A 20-gauge Chiba type needle is introduced into the posterior aspect of the lesion. Note needle tip (*arrow*). (*E*) Small amount of absolute alcohol rapidly diffuses throughout the lesion with injection, which appears as an echogenic region in the mid-to-posterior aspect of the lesion. (*F*) After injection of ethanol, RFA is performed that also demonstrates an echogenic response within the lesion and surrounding tissue. (*G*) After the procedure, arterial phase contrast-enhanced CT scan demonstrates area of decreased density in the region of the mass with normal-appearing hyperemic rim of contrast enhancement (*arrow*). Patient also had minimal bibasilar atelectases and small amount of subcapsular fluid and blood.

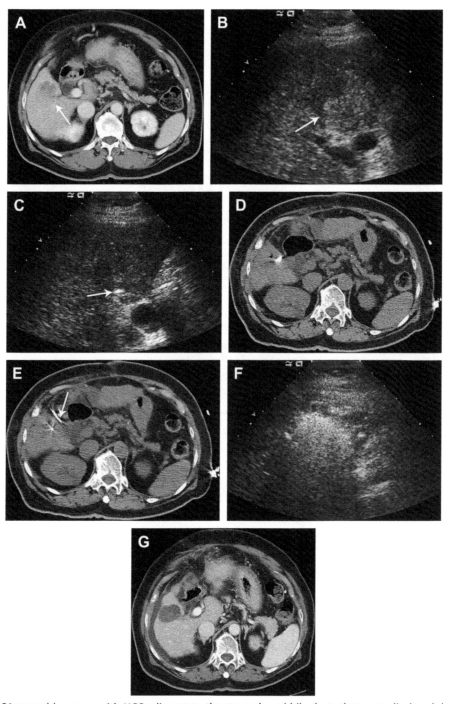

Fig. 5. An 81-year-old woman with HCC adjacent to the stomach and bile ducts that were displaced during RFA using hydrodissection. (*A*) CT scan demonstrates portion of mass (*arrow*) adjacent to the pylorus and common bile duct. (*B*) Ultrasound image demonstrates isoechoic well-encapsulated mass (*arrow*). (*C*) RF needle tip (*arrow*) is identified being placed into the mass. (*D*) Location of needle is checked with CT and demonstrates needle in close proximity to the pylorus. (*E*) This image demonstrates RF needle and blunt-tip needle (*arrow*) after infusion of D5W to displace the pylorus and the common bile duct from the RFA needle site. (*F*) Echogenic response after RFA. (*G*) Twelve-hour CT scan after RFA demonstrates area of decreased density in the liver corresponding to RFA site. There was no injury to the pylorus.

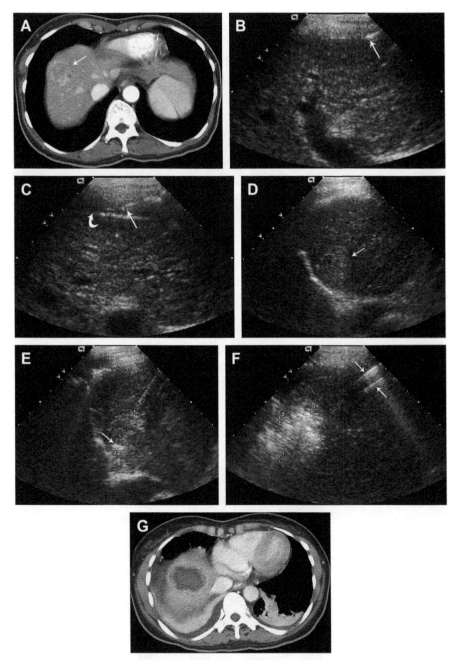

Fig. 6. A 52-year-old woman with large HCC at the dome of the liver. Scan demonstrates use of artificial ascites and switchbox technique. (*A*) Contrast-enhanced CT scan demonstrates fairly large lesion at the dome of the liver (*arrow*). (*B*) High-resolution ultrasound of the anterior liver demonstrates needle (*arrow*) placed at the liver capsule (*arrow*). (*C*) There is infusion of D5W with the needle, and a catheter (*arrow*) is positioned over the liver capsule (*curved arrow*). This catheter is placed toward the dome of the liver to create artificial ascites between the liver lesion and the diaphragm. (*D*) Ultrasound examination demonstrates large echogenic lesion abutting the dome of the diaphragm (*arrow*). (*E*) Ultrasound image demonstrates tip of the RF needle within the lesion (*arrow*). (*F*) Note two needles positioned into the lesion (*arrow*) for application of RFA. There is creation of a large echogenic region (*calipers*). (*G*) Immediate follow-up contrast CT scan demonstrates large area of decreased density corresponding to region of RFA toward the dome. Note the artificial ascites surrounding the liver and bilateral atelectases and pleural effusions.

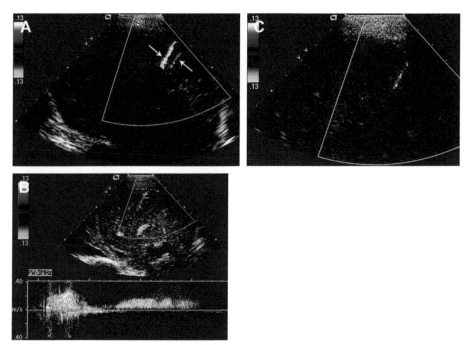

Fig. 7. A 52-year-old woman after RFA with two needles. This is the same case as illustrated in **Fig. 6** demonstrating the "patent track" sign. (*A*) Color flow demonstrates two-color track to the liver surface (*arrow*). (*B*) Doppler demonstrates that the track corresponded to venous fistula to the surface of the liver. (*C*) Within 3 minutes after probe pressure, one of these fistulas spontaneously closed, and within 5 minutes, both fistulas closed. This scan demonstrates the advantage of ultrasound to demonstrate potential complications that may occur even with RFA.

therapy with systemic or regional chemotherapy or radiotherapy or chemoembolization can be considered at this point. Serum or biochemical tumor markers may be assessed after treatment. This approach is especially helpful in patients with elevated markers, such as alpha fetoprotein, to see if they have become elevated, which could indicate tumor recurrence or development of a new HCC. CT, MRI, or, less frequently, sonography may be used to evaluate the results of therapy. We usually perform these modalities immediately after treatment and at regular 3-month intervals for 1 year, 6-month intervals for another year, and then again 1 year after that. If there are other significant risk factors, such hepatitis C, then CT or MRI every 3 months may be considered.

METHODS OF TREATMENT
Combined Therapy

RFA may be used alone or in combination with other methods for treatment of renal and liver tumors (**Box 1**). For instance, different local agents such as absolute alcohol or acetic acid may be injected coaxially or with an individual needle for combined therapy with RFA. RFA could be combined with hepatic resection, treating a lesion in one segment of the liver and resecting it in another lesion. RFA also may be used in conjunction with systemic chemotherapy at the time of ablation and multiple catheter-based technologies. A few of these different therapies are described later.

Percutaneous Ethanol Injection Therapy

PEI therapy (PEIT) has been used for ablation of focal tumors, especially HCC, in Japan.[5,6] Alcohol causes tissue destruction by intracellular diffusion, dehydration of intercellular proteins, and consequent coagulation necrosis. HCCs are uniquely suited for PEIT, whereas other tumors, such as liver metastases, have less favorable results. This is because liver metastases, such as colorectal masses, are usually firm, and firmness does not allow dispersion of ethanol. HCCs are hypervascular and have a softer consistency, however, which allows easier distribution of ethanol. Research has shown that ethanol alone has been effective in the treatment of small HCCs. Lencioni and colleagues[11] compared PEI to RFA in treatments of HCCs. They demonstrated the 1- and 2-year local recurrent survival rates of 98% and 96%,

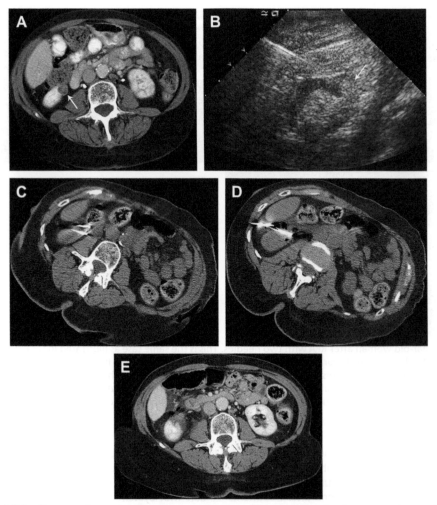

Fig. 8. Renal RFA of lower pole renal cell carcinoma using RFA and hydrodissection in same patient as **Fig. 3.** (*A*) CT scan demonstrates a second solid mass on the inferior pole of right kidney (*arrow*). Also note that the large bowel lies directly over this mass. (*B*) Ultrasound guidance of RF needle being placed into lower pole lesion (*arrow*). (*C*) CT scan was used to demonstrate satisfactory position of needle and lower pole lesion and demonstrate placement of blunted tipped needle adjacent to the large bowel, in which there is infusion of D5W (anterior needle). (*D*) With continued infusion of water and continuous RFA, there is evidence of microbubble formations surrounding the lesion and increasing the distance between the RF needle tip and the colon. (*E*) Follow-up CT of lesion 2 demonstrates avascular region corresponding to RFA site. Also note evidence of water displacing the colon from the lesion even on this 6-hour follow-up CT scan.

respectively, for RFA versus 83% and 62%, respectively, in which PEI was used alone. The 1- and 2-year event-free survival rates were 86% and 64%, respectively, for the RFA group and 77% and 43%, respectively, for the PEI group. This was in a comparison of patients treated with HCC with RFA alone versus PEI.

Others have described the use of PEIT in combination with RFA. It may be used as a fairly powerful technique, because PEIT and RFA cause tissue ablation by different mechanisms. After PEIT there may be decreased blood flow to the tumor and less heat sink effect with RFA. Zhang and

colleagues[12] evaluated patients with HCC treated with radiofrequency alone or combined radiofrequency and PEI. In their results, they found 1-, 2-, 3-, 4-, and 5-year overall survival rates for RFA plus PEI of 95%, 89%, 76%, 63%, and 49%, respectively, compared with RFA alone group, in which survival rates were 90%, 69%, 58%, 50%, and 36%, respectively. They felt it was a statistically significant survival curve for the RFA plus PEI group, with a survival rate significantly better than for the RFA alone group. They noted that for tumors smaller than 3 cm, however, survival with RFA alone was similar to that of RFA

Box 1
Combined therapies with radiofrequency ablation

Local

    Ethanol

    Acetic acid

    Saline

Resection

External beam radiation

Systemic chemotherapy

Catheter-based techniques

    Chemoembolization

    Bland embolization

    Infusion therapy

    Radioembolization

    Drug-eluting microspheres

---

plus PEI. For tumors between 3.1 and 5 cm, the RFA plus PEI performed better than RFA alone (see **Fig. 4**).[12]

Embolization Techniques

Several different articles have discussed different chemoembolization techniques, which vary from bland embolization to chemoembolization with different chemotherapeutic agents, to focal radiation therapy using yttrium microspheres. The combination of use of transarterial chemoembolization plus RFA has been advocated for use for certain tumors. Historically, the first RFA in a renal tumor described in radiology literature used the combination of catheter embolization to decrease blood flow followed by RFA to successfully ablate renal cell carcinoma.[13] Likewise, several researchers have advocated combined chemoembolization and RFA for larger hepatomas to increase tumor necrosis. This research has included different studies looking at different transcatheter embolization techniques combined with RFA. These studies are too numerous to review in detail.

One of these studies was by Lencioni and colleagues,[14] in which they used combined therapy of doxorubicin-eluting beads plus RFA. They found that the volume of induced necrosis as measured on imaging increased from 4.8 cm after RFA to 7.5 cm after doxorubicin-eluting beads administration, which is an increase of 61%. They felt that intra-arterial doxorubicin-eluting bead administration substantially enhanced the effect of RFA alone. Likewise, several clinical trials demonstrated that the combined effect of chemoembolization plus RFA is superior in improving survival of patients with HCC larger than 3 cm compared with transarterial chemoembolization alone or RFA alone. For instance, in a study by Cheng and colleagues,[15] the rate of objective response sustained for at least 6 months was highest for the transarterial chemoembolization RFA group at 54%, compared with either transarterial chemoembolization alone at 35% or RFA alone at 36%.[14]

Radiofrequency Electrocautery

In 1990, McGahan and colleagues[7] published a report on the concept of percutaneous ablation of liver tissue using radiofrequency electrocautery. This concept was novel because of proposed use of focal application of RF energy in an animal liver using ultrasound guidance. A monopolar electrode with an insulated distal tip was placed into liver tissue, and tissue coagulation was observed. Subsequently, several different methods of increasing tissue ablation have been developed, including combination of therapies such as PEIT and chemoembolization with RFA. Some initial results of RFA in the liver were promising; others' results were disappointing. With more recent technical developments in RF energy, delivery, and development of new and different needles, use of RFA alone has shown fairly good results. In a study by Lencioni and colleagues,[16] patients with early cirrhosis, such as a CHILD's class A cirrhosis, with a solitary HCC treated by RFA alone had fairly high 1-, 3-, and 5-year survival rates of 100%, 89%, and 69%, respectively. The best response was for tumors less than or equal to 3 cm in diameter.[16]

Although there is fairly good response with early-stage cirrhosis and HCC, the response for metastatic disease has been shown to be less favorable. For instance, in a study by Abdalla and colleagues[17] in patients with colorectal liver metastases, the overall recurrence was most common after RFA alone (84%), versus 64% when RFA was used in conjunction with resection, versus 53% when resection alone was used. Overall survival rate was highest after resection, with a 4-year survival rate after resection alone of 65%, compared with 36% survival rate at 4 years with RFA plus resection, and only a 22% 4-year survival rate with RFA alone.[17]

Postablative Management

Postablative syndrome is a flu-like syndrome that lasts from 1 to 3 days but can last longer. Patients have general malaise and may have flu-like symptoms that may persist as long as 2 weeks.

Occasionally patients run a low-grade fever. If the fever persists or spikes, superimposed infection should be excluded. Often patients' fever or flu-like symptoms are in proportion to the number of ablations and tumor size. Pain also may occur after ablation, especially in patients with subcapsular lesions.

COMPLICATIONS

Probably the largest series to date demonstrating the complications of RFA is a series published by Livraghi and colleagues,[18] in which they surveyed 41 Italian centers that perform percutaneous RFA as part of a collaborative group to evaluate associated complications rate. Complete response was achieved in only 70% of all tumors. The mortality rate was 0.3%, with a complication rate of 2.2%. The most frequent complications included peritoneal hemorrhage, neoplastic seeding, intrahepatic abscess, and intestinal perforation. Minor complications were observed in less than 5% of patients. Because this trial included 2320 patients with 3554 lesions and was performed in a multicenter fashion by different physicians, it attests to the fact that RFA is a relatively low-risk procedure for treatment of focal liver tumors.

DIFFICULT REGIONS

Several difficult regions in either the liver or the gallbladder may decrease tumor necrosis or increase potential complications. Some of these areas include lesions abutting the diaphragm or pericardium, lesions adjacent to structures such as the bowel or gallbladder, or more central lesions adjacent to large vessels or major bile ducts or ureter (**Box 2**). For these difficult regions, many different methods may be used to displace the diaphragm, the bowel, or ureter from the tumor (see **Figs. 5** and **8**), including use of hydrodissection using dextrose in water. Others have advocated a balloon placed between the lesion and the organ, such as between the liver and colon. Hydroperfusion using cooled D5W injected into the bile ducts or ureter may help prevent injury. For treatment of HCC adjacent to the gallbladder, ethanol may be used to prevent gallbladder injury (**Box 3**).

Diaphragm

The diaphragm may be a more difficult area in which to treat focal liver masses. There have been reports of abscesses leading to sepsis, biliary-broncho fistulas, and cardiac tamponade. This has been caused by nonvisualized "tines" that have been placed inadvertently into the

diaphragm or the pericardium. There also has been some question of increasing pain if RFA is performed close to the diaphragm. An article by Head and colleagues[19] discussed 29 patients in whom they used expandable electrodes to perform RFA with conscious sedation in liver lesions next to the diaphragm. If the patients had shoulder pain, the needle was pulled back. The authors noted, however, that of the 29 patients, 5 had pain, 1 had severe pain, and 4 had mild pain.

In a different article by Kang and colleagues,[20] they evaluated two groups of patients: 31 patients who had lesion abutting the diaphragm and 49 patients with lesions above the portal vein but not touching the diaphragm. They noted no complications in the performance of RFA in patients with lesions abutting the diaphragm; however, they did note difference in tumor ablation rate between HCCs abutting the diaphragm versus HCCs below the diaphragm. In patients who had HCCs below the diaphragm, they had a 98% success rate, compared with 84% initial success rate with lesions abutting the diaphragm. They had local progression of disease—short time periods in 29% of lesions abutting the diaphragm.[20] Also noted in the series by Kang and colleagues was the use of a nonexpandable but cooled tip needle, with which they noted some

---

Box 2
Difficult regions

Diaphragm

Pericardium (heart)

Gallbladder

Major bile ducts

Large vessels

Central lesions

Ureter

Box 3
Difficult regions: maneuvers

Hydrodissection: D5W

Balloon interposition

Ethanol ablation

Hydroperfusion (cooling)

   Bile ducts

   Ureter

Others

diaphragmatic swelling in lesions abutting the diaphragm but no major complications or pain. They did observe hemothorax in one patient and a pleural effusion in one patient, however.

There has been some discussion of whether different techniques should be used to decrease potential pain in diaphragmatic lesions. Some of these techniques have included inserting water or D5W between the diaphragm and the lesion, inserting D5W above the diaphragm and the lesion, dropping the lung when RFA is performed with CT or laparoscopically. In general, Teratani and colleagues[21] felt that it is important to use a cooled-tip rather than expandable electrode for lesions adjacent to the diaphragm and watch the echogenic response. If the echogenicity progresses to the diaphragm, then the RFA ablation could be stopped. They felt that the use of D5W to separate the liver from the diaphragm may be helpful to decrease complications. RFA with the assistance of artificial ascites is a simple and safe technique for treatment of hepatic dome tumors abutting the diaphragm. The use of dextrose (5%) in water (D5W) is ideal because it is nonionic in nature. This technique allows the liver to be displaced from the diaphragm, which helps prevent thermal injury to the diaphragm and may allow better visualization of the tumor by ultrasound (see **Fig. 6**).

Peritoneal adhesions and tumors located in the bare area are limitations to the applications of this technique, however. This technique may be performed via several methods. It can include needle positioning into the liver during inspiration, which is removed slightly during expiration so that it lies on top of the liver capsule. D5W can be gently injected over the liver capsule, and once enough solution is observed, a guidewire or small catheter can be placed above the liver capsule. The catheter can be placed in the region of the tumor for installation of D5W. Kondo and colleagues[22] in 2006 also advocated artificial ascites in RFA of the liver for cancers adjacent to the gastrointestinal tract. They inserted from 250 mL to more than 3 L of D5W to separate the bowel from the liver lesion. They were 78% successful in separating bowel from the liver lesion. In their series, they had one bowel injury, which was thought to be secondary to bowel adhesions.

Gallbladder

Chopra and colleagues[23] felt that RFA adjacent to the gallbladder was a safe procedure; however, 75% of their patients who had RFA adjacent to the gallbladder had immediate pain. The pain lasted from 5 to 21 days. Fifty percent of patients had fever. No patients experienced death or cholecystectomy. More recently in an animal model, Lee and colleagues[24] demonstrated that if an RF needle is placed perpendicular to the lumen of the gallbladder, it should be at least 1 cm away from the gallbladder lumen. If it is placed parallel to the gallbladder lumen, there is a high probability that there could be either acute injury or delayed bile leak with injury to the gallbladder. As such, they advocate other methods for RFA of lesions adjacent to the gallbladder. We believe that gallbladder injury is a real risk. In these lesions, we would perform combination therapy for larger lesions, including ethanol ablation of lesions adjacent to the gallbladder, with RFA of the lesion more removed from the gallbladder (see **Fig. 4**). We would approach the lesion so that the needle is placed perpendicular to the gallbladder rather than parallel to the gallbladder, ensuring a margin of safety between the liver lesion and the gallbladder to prevent thermal injury.

Kidney

RFA for the kidney is similar to RFA for the liver. Site-specific differentiations in therapy must be considered, however, including anterior tumors adjacent to organs such as the large bowel. Similar hydrodissection would be used as discussed for RFA of the liver. Upper-pole tumors may be treated with the patient in the prone position using anangled technique, with guidance either by ultrasound or CT. McGahan and colleagues[25] proposed use of RFA of upper-pole lesions with patients in the supine position and using a transhepatic approach (see **Fig. 3**). For larger tumors, clustered probes, overlapping ablations, or switchbox technique may be used. For tumors near the ureter, hydrodissection and chilled D5W placed into the ureter via stent may be helpful to prevent injury. In general, exophytic lesions smaller than 3 cm are most amenable to complete tumor ablation using RFA.

There has been some discussion concerning the role of either fine needle aspiration biopsy or core biopsy of lesions within the kidney.[26,27] In general, fine needle aspiration technique may prove to be superior to core biopsy in the kidney.[26,27] Different series have had different results concerning the rate of benign versus malignant lesions within the kidney. For instance, in a study by Beland and colleagues,[26] renal biopsy was diagnostic in 90% of the cases with approximately a quarter of the lesions being benign. Not all of these biopsies were performed before RFA. In another publication by Heilbrun and colleagues,[27] however, only 5% of all lesions underwent CT-guided biopsy before treatment with percutaneous RFA proved to be benign. Ninety-five percent of lesions in which there was satisfactory retrieval of cells were malignant lesions.

In a publication by Gervais and colleagues,[28] the results of RFA for renal tumors were good for small lesions. They noted 100% complete necrosis of tumors smaller than 3 cm, 92% complete necrosis in tumors 3 to 5 cm, and only a 25% complete necrosis rate in tumors larger than 5 cm. In another article by Zagoria and colleagues,[29] they found a 93% complete necrosis rate at follow-up of 13 months with 100% of lesions, with complete necrosis when the lesion was 3.7 cm or only 71% necrosis rate in lesions larger than 3.7 cm. Best results with renal RFA are in tumors that were exophytic rather than more central tumors.

Many of the RFA treatments in the kidneys are guided by CT; however, in our practice we use ultrasound for initial needle placement and use CT to check final needle placement. This has the advantage of using sonography for real-time needle placement without the use of radiation. CT is helpful to ensure that the needle is not in close proximity to surrounding bowel or ureter. If there is close proximity to the surrounding bowel, a similar technique has been advocated with RFA of the liver adjacent to the bowel. This includes the use of artificial ascites or hydrodissection. The needle is placed into the renal cell carcinoma, and another needle with a blunted tip is placed between the lesion and the bowel. Artificial ascites is then injected using dextrose (5%) in water (D5W) to displace the overlying bowel from the kidney (see **Fig. 8**). This has been a helpful technique for preventing injuries to overlying bowel. Likewise, injuries to the ureter have occurred with RFA.

In analyzing complications from RFA of the kidney, the main complication seems to be ureteric injury. In 100 lesions treated by Gervais and colleagues,[28] there were two ureteric injuries and one urine leak. As such, cryoablation has been advocated as a safer method than percutaneous RFA. In a publication by Littrup and colleagues,[30] they reported a 6% major complication rate and a 22% minor complication rate. They also reported one ureteric stricture in 49 cryoablations performed in their series.

Different techniques have been used to prevent ureteric injuries, including use of artificial ascites to displace the lesion from the ureter. This approach may be more difficult, however, because both of these structures are fairly fixed in the retroperitoneum. Other techniques have included installation of cooled D5W into the ureter to prevent ureteric injury. Protection of the ureter during RFA of renal cell carcinoma includes retrograde pyeloperfusion with cooled dextrose 5% in water.[31]

SUMMARY

Ultrasound alone can be used to guide treatment of many hepatic tumors. In the kidney, combination of ultrasound and CT is often used. Ultrasound may be used for needle placement, whereas CT is used to identify vital structures that may overlie the treated lesion, such as the ureter or adjacent bowel. Several different technical factors must be mastered before performing RFA in the abdomen to minimize complications and maximize results.

ACKNOWLEDGMENTS

Special thanks to Angela Zabel for typing the manuscript.

REFERENCES

1. Tabuse K. A new operative procedure of hepatic surgery using a microwave tissue coagulator. Nippon Geka Hokan 1979;48(2):160–72.
2. Seki T, Wakabayashi M, Nakagawa T, et al. Ultrasonically guided percutaneous microwave coagulation therapy for small hepatocellular carcinoma. Cancer 1994;74(3):817–25.
3. Hashimoto D, Takami M, Idesuki Y. In depth radiation therapy Nd:YAG laser for malignant tumors of the liver under ultrasonic imaging. Gastroenterology 1985;88:A1663.
4. Onik GM, Atkinson D, Zemel R, et al. Cryosurgery of liver cancer. Semin Surg Oncol 1993;9(4):309–17.
5. Livraghi T, Salmi A, Bolondi L, et al. Small hepatocellular carcinoma: percutaneous alcohol injection. Results in 23 patients. Radiology 1988;168(2):313–7.
6. Shiina S, Tagawa K, Unuma T, et al. Percutaneous ethanol injection therapy of hepatocellular carcinoma: analysis of 77 patients. Am J Roentgenol 1990;155(6):1221–6.
7. McGahan JP, Browning PD, Brock JM, et al. Hepatic ablation using radiofrequency electrocautery. Invest Radiol 1990;25(3):267–70.
8. Goldberg SN, Gazelle GS, Dawson SL, et al. Tissue ablation with radiofrequency using multiprobe arrays. Acad Radiol 1995;2(8):670–4.
9. Lorentzen T. A cooled needle electrode for radiofrequency tissue ablation: thermodynamic aspects of improved performance compared with conventional needle design. Acad Radiol 1995;3(7):556–63.
10. Gili IS, Hsu TH, Fox RL, et al. Laparoscopic and percutaneous radiofrequency ablation of the kidney: acute and chronic porcine study. Urology 2000; 56(2):197–200.

11. Lencioni RA, Allgaier HP, Cioni D, et al. Small hepatocellular carcinoma in cirrhosis: randomized comparison of radio-frequency thermal ablation versus percutaneous ethanol injection. Radiology 2003;228(1):235–40.

12. Zhang YJ, Liang HH, Chen MS, et al. Hepatocellular carcinoma treated with radiofrequency ablation with or without ethanol injection: a prospective randomized trial. Radiology 2007;244(2):599–607.

13. Hall WH, McGahan JP, Link DP, et al. Combined embolization and percutaneous radiofrequency ablation of a solid renal tumor. Am J Roentgenol 2000;174(6):1592–4.

14. Lencioni R, Crocetti L, Petruzzi P, et al. Doxorubicineluting bead-enhanced radiofrequency ablation of hepatocellular carcinoma: a pilot clinical study. J Hepatol 2008;49(2):217–22.

15. Cheng BQ, Jia CQ, Liu CT, et al. Chemoembolization combined with radiofrequency ablation for patients with hepatocellular carcinoma larger than 3 cm: a randomized controlled trial. JAMA 2008;299(14): 1669–77.

16. Lencioni R, Cioni D, Crocetti L, et al. Early-stage hepatocellular carcinoma in patients with cirrhosis: long-term results of percutaneous image-guided radiofrequency ablation. Radiology 2005;234(3): 961–7.

17. Abdalla EK, Vauthey JN, Ellis LM, et al. Recurrence and outcomes following hepatic resection, radiofrequency ablation, and combined resection/ablation for colorectal liver metastases. Ann Surg 2004; 239(6):818–25.

18. Livraghi T, Solbiati L, Meloni MF, et al. Treatment of focal liver tumors with percutaneous radiofrequency ablation: complications encountered in a multicenter study. Radiology 2003;226(2):441–51.

19. Head HW, Dodd GD III, Dalrymple NC, et al. Percutaneous radiofrequency ablation of hepatic tumors against the diaphragm: frequency of diaphragmatic injury. Radiology 2007;243(3):877–84.

20. Kang TW, Rhim H, Kim EY, et al. Percutaneous radiofrequency ablation for hepatocellular carcinoma abutting the diaphragm: assessment of safety and therapeutic efficacy [abstract SSQ08-04]. In: Programs and Abstracts of the 93rd Scientific Assembly and Annual Meeting of the Radiological Society of North America. Chicago; November 25–30, 2007. p. 579.

21. Teratani T, Yoshida H, Shiina S, et al. Radiofrequency ablation for hepatocellular carcinoma in so-called high-risk locations. Hepatology 2006;43(5):1101–8.

22. Kondo Y, Yoshida H, Shiina S, et al. Artificial ascites technique for percutaneous radiofrequency ablation of liver cancer adjacent to the gastrointestinal tract. Br J Surg 2006;93(10):1277–82.

23. Chopra S, Dodd GD III, Chanin MP, et al. Radiofrequency ablation of hepatic tumors adjacent to the gallbladder: feasibility and safety. Am J Roentgenol 2003;180(3):697–701.

24. Lee J, Rhim H, Jeon YH, et al. Radiofrequency ablation of liver adjacent to body of gallbladder: histopathologic changes of gallbladder wall in pig model. Am J Roentgenol 2008;190:418–25.

25. McGahan JP, Ro KM, Evans CP, et al. Efficacy of transhepatic radiofrequency ablation of renal cell carcinoma. Am J Roentgenol 2006;186(5):S311–5.

26. Beland MD, Mayo-Smith WW, Dupuy DE, et al. Diagnostic yield of 58 consecutive imaging-guided biopsies of solid renal masses: should we biopsy all that are indeterminate? Am J Roentgenol 2007;188: 792–7.

27. Heilbrun ME, Zagoria RJ, Garvin AJ, et al. CT-guided biopsy for the diagnosis of renal tumors before treatment with percutaneous ablation. Am J Roentgenol 2007;188(6):1500–5.

28. Gervais DA, McGovern FJ, Arellano RS, et al. Radiofrequency ablation of renal cell carcinoma: Part 1. Indications, results, and role in patient management over a 6-year period and ablation of 100 tumors. Am J Roentgenol 2005;185(1):64–71.

29. Zagoria RJ, Traver MA, Werle DM, et al. Oncologic efficacy of CT-guided percutaneous radiofrequency ablation of renal cell carcinomas. Am J Roentgenol 2007;189(2):429–36.

30. Littrup PJ, Ahmed A, Aoun HD, et al. CT-guided percutaneous cryotherapy of renal masses. J Vasc Interv Radiol 2007;18(3):383–92.

31. Cantwell CP, Wah TM, Gervais DA, et al. Protecting the ureter during radiofrequency ablation of renal cell cancer: a pilot study of retrograde pyeloperfusion with cooled dextrose 5% in water. J Vasc Interv Radiol 2008;19(7):1034–40.

Pelvic Drainage: Image Guidance and Technique

Carol L. Phillips, BSc, MBBS, MRCS, FRCSC[a], Petra L. Williams, BSc, MBBS, MRCP[a],
Anthony F. Watkinson, BSc, MSc (oxon), MBBS, FRCS, FRCR[a,b],*

KEYWORDS

- Pelvic drainage • Ultrasound • Abscess
- Percutaneous • Endocavitary

Management of pelvic abscesses and collections can be challenging in terms of their localization and subsequent access for purposes of aspiration or drainage. Although formerly the territory of surgeons, improvements in imaging technology and applied techniques now enable interventional radiologists to perform percutaneous or endocavitary drainage of even the most difficult abscesses. By employing such minimally invasive methods, treatment has become faster, cheaper, less painful, and more acceptable to the patient, making it the option of choice. Various combinations of imaging modality and route of access can be used depending on the location of the abscess, individual patient constraints, and operator preference. Although CT provides accurate localization and drain placement, ultrasound is becoming increasingly used through its continually developing technology. This proficiency, together with the lack of ionizing radiation, real-time imaging, and portability of the equipment, allows pelvic drainage to be safely performed in children as well as adults, repeated if necessary, and performed in various settings, including intensive care units. This article focuses on the different ultrasound-guided techniques used for pelvic drainage, including difficult access, and, equally important, discusses when it is not appropriate.

INDICATIONS FOR PELVIC DRAINAGE

The obvious indication for pelvic drainage is a symptomatic abscess, particularly in patients who have uncontrolled pain, sepsis, or signs of local obstruction. The abscess source can vary and include enteric, intramuscular, tubo-ovarian, or prostatic origins, and often develops as a postoperative complication. A percutaneous or endocavitary technique is acceptable in patients in whom no other reason for surgery is indicated. If the fluid collection is demonstrated to be purulent, attempted aspiration is incomplete, or a communication with bowel is suspected, catheter drainage is recommended. Furthermore, drainage can be a useful adjunct before more formal surgical treatment, particularly in cases of periappendiceal or peridiverticular abscesses, when the patient's clinical condition can be optimized and the number of two-stage operations can potentially be reduced.[1,2] Noninfected collections such as loculated ascites, hematomas, and lymphoceles can be aspirated, drained, or even treated with sclerosants in refractory cases. The simplest indication is acquisition of a diagnostic specimen before embarking on more definitive treatment.

GENERAL CONTRAINDICATIONS

Fortunately, general contraindications are relatively few and mainly involve issues surrounding coagulopathy that are not correctable and the uncooperative patient. In the presence of acute peritonitis or large volumes of free fluid or gas, the patient may be better proceeding to surgery unless they are deemed unfit. Nevertheless, some patients may benefit from percutaneous drainage and optimization of their condition before proceeding to definitive surgery.

[a] Department of Clinical Imaging, Royal Devon and Exeter NHS Foundation Trust, Barrack Road, Exeter, Devon, EX2 5DW, UK
[b] The Peninsula Medical School, Barrack Road, Exeter, Devon, EX2 5DW, UK
* Corresponding author.
E-mail address: anthony.watkinson@rdeft.nhs.uk (A.F. Watkinson).

Ultrasound Clin 4 (2009) 73–81
doi:10.1016/j.cult.2009.03.003

If there is doubt regarding the nature of a collection, an initial aspiration for microbial culture is advised before deciding definitive treatment. Percutaneous aspiration alone is contraindicated for definitive treatment of collections where there is a connection to the bowel or urinary tract.

Method-specific contraindications are discussed further under each of the following procedure headings.

GENERAL TECHNIQUES: SELDINGER AND TROCAR

Two accepted methods of catheter placement are described. They each have their own advantages and disadvantages. It is important to take this into consideration when planning a pelvic drainage, because one technique will be more suitable than the other depending on the individual aspects of the clinical situation. Both methods require the use of strict aseptic technique by the operator and a full sterile field, including gown as well as gloves, and patient drapes should be standard practice.

Trocar

This technique uses a catheter that is directly mounted onto a sharp-tipped stylet or trocar. The catheter can be inserted into the abscess adjacent to a guide needle that has been already placed following sterilization and local anesthesia of the skin. Positioning of the guide needle is important because it allows safe passage of the trocar in an immediately parallel direction. A small-bore needle is adequate, but the length needs to be calculated depending on the depth of the abscess to allow enough of the needle to sit externally and act as a visual aid to trocar placement. Accuracy with regards to the path and angle of the trocar can still be achieved despite respiratory or other motion by the patient. Once a satisfactory position of the guide needle is obtained, a small skin incision and blunt dissection adjacent to the needle entry point are performed before insertion of the trocar and catheter. The catheter is then advanced into the abscess while simultaneously withdrawing the trocar (**Fig. 1**A–D).

Advantages include the rapidity of the technique as a result of the reduced number of steps involved and reduced leakage of abscess contents along the track during dilator or catheter changes.

This method is of benefit to all patients, particularly pediatric patients who require sedation or even general anesthesia, for whom the time involved can be decreased to a minimum, making the procedure even safer. Disadvantages are few

and involve problems with repositioning a catheter that has been initially incorrectly sited.

Seldinger

First described in 1952 as a method for obtaining angiographic access, this technique is now widely employed during many interventional procedures, including abscess drainage.[3] Following sterilization and local anesthesia of the skin, a hollow needle is inserted into the abscess cavity under ultrasound guidance, followed by a guidewire that is small enough to fit through the lumen of the needle. The needle is then withdrawn, a small skin incision is made, and a catheter is placed over the wire left in situ, which is then removed once satisfactory catheter position has been obtained. In general, an 18-G angiographic needle is suitable for a 0.035- or 0.038-in guidewire and placement of an 8 to 14F catheter (depending on abscess location and viscosity of contents). Alternatively, a 21- or 22-G needle can be inserted, which will accommodate a 0.018-in wire, but requires subsequent dilatation of the tract and exchange for a 0.035-in wire before catheter placement. The larger catheter bores may require sequential dilators to aid introduction (**Fig. 2**A–D).

The advantage of this technique is the ability to manipulate and place the wire in the exact location required for final catheter positioning. Disadvantages mainly involve the time required to complete the multiple steps of the process, problems with wire kinking, and leakage from around the wire during removal of the needle or dilators. The latter can lead to spillage of infected or malignant contents into adjacent tissues and also decompression of smaller collections, making catheter placement more difficult.

ANATOMIC CONSIDERATIONS

Whichever method and route of access are chosen to perform pelvic drainage, a thorough knowledge of the anatomy is essential so that safe catheter deployment and subsequent management can be achieved. The operator should be very clear about the abscess location, immediate anatomic structures, and those in the potential pathway of the needle. If the procedure is to be performed under ultrasound guidance, it is essential that the abscess or collection can be clearly identified along with the surrounding or intervening structures.

In addition, the differences between pelvic organs of the male and female and in children need to be recognized because this can influence the planning of the procedure. Theoretically, traversing any pelvic structure during drainage or

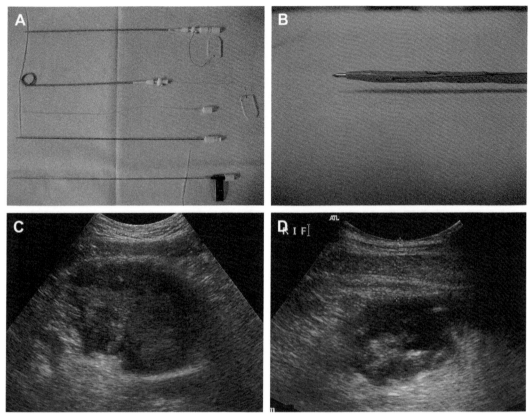

Fig. 1. (*A*) Catheter set for trocar use (top of image), with the individual catheter components (pigtail catheter, plastic and metal stiffeners, trocar needle) shown below it. (*B*) The trocar needle at the catheter tip. (*C*) Transabdominal ultrasound image demonstrating complex pelvic collection of mixed echogenicity. (*D*) Subsequent image. After insertion of pigtail drain and aspiration of thick pus, the collection has reduced in size. The catheter was left on free drainage.

aspiration should be avoided, particularly the colon and blood vessels for obvious reasons; however, there is the rare occasion when an inter-loop abscess will be accessed by transgressing the small bowel and aspirating it to dryness using a small-bore needle. These situations arise in Crohn's patients for whom the lifetime possibility of surgery is high and therefore avoided if possible.

Anatomy of the pelvis can be divided into extra- and intraperitoneal structures, with the colon and bladder constituting the extraperitoneal structures and the small bowel and neurovascular structures lying truly intraperitoneally. The remaining pelvic organs are closely related to the peritoneum itself, which covers the anterior aspect of the rectum and then folds to create either the rectovesical pouch (males) or pouch of Douglas (females) before continuing over the superior aspect of the uterus or bladder anteriorly (**Fig. 3**). The prostate and seminal vesicles in the male lie more deeply in the true pelvis, at the base of the bladder. Abscesses and collections commonly develop in

the pelvis, even when the source is within the abdomen, because it is the most gravity-dependent part. In addition, there are potential spaces which encourage abscess formation: the recto-vesical pouch and pouch of Douglas (both intra-peritoneal) and the space of Retzius (retropubic or prevesical space), which is extraperitoneal and can therefore communicate with the retroperito-neal space, anterior abdominal wall, and femoral sheath, leading to potential infection spread.

Unless the abscess or collection is easily visible with an ultrasound probe, a predrainage planning CT is advisable to assess the anatomy.

PATIENT PREPARATION

Most pre-procedure preparations are common to all methods, with some variations depending on the individual patient. All patients require a coag-ulation and hemodynamics screen within the previous 24 hours. Prophylactic antibiotic admin-istration is also essential, although the majority

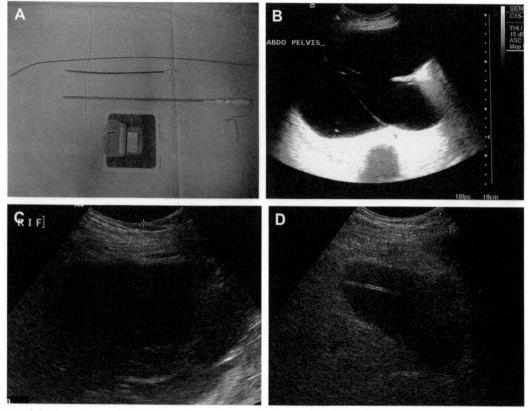

Fig. 2. (*A*) Image demonstrates the supplementary equipment required (in addition to needle and catheter) for delivery of a catheter with the Seldinger technique: a short stiff wire, dilator, and drain fix. (*B*) Image demonstrates the guidewire correctly positioned within a collection before overwire catheter insertion. (*C*) Tranasaxial ultrasound image demonstrating an infected collection in the right adnexal region. (*D*) Subsequent image (longitudinal view) demonstrates the dual echogenic lines of the catheter within the collection.

of patients will already be receiving them. Informed written consent from the patient or parent/guardian (for the child or mentally incapacitated adult) is obtained by the interventional radiologist performing the procedure. Some routes of access will require the adult patient to be sedated, and children certainly need appropriate sedation, which reduces the anxiety levels and pain response and ensures that the patient remains cooperative during the procedure. The level of sedation can be tailored to the individual, ranging from light sedation to full general anesthetic, the latter being necessary in the very young.[4] Consequently, anesthetic support and full resuscitative equipment are required. Furthermore, the environment for pediatric cases must be kept warm to avoid loss of body heat. Ultrasound-guided drainage means that there are no concerns with regards to radiation exposure, reducing time constraints and allowing repetition of the procedure should this be necessary.

ROUTES OF ACCESS: PERCUTANEOUS AND ENDOCAVITARY

All established routes of access can be classed as percutaneous (transabdominal, transgluteal, and transperineal) or endocavitary (transrectal and transvaginal). Each method is described and their individual applications discussed when used in conjunction with ultrasound in the following sections.

Percutaneous: Transabdominal

This route is the most commonly employed and well-established method used for percutaneous drainage, particularly because the supine position required is practical, even in the most acutely unwell patients. Nevertheless, safely accessing the pelvis via this route is not as straightforward as the abdomen, and the most common problem encountered is the small bowel which lies anteriorly. The bladder poses a less common problem because it can be decompressed with a urinary

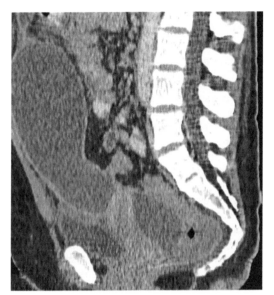

Fig. 3. Sagittal CT reformat demonstrates loculated peritoneal fluid collection, with fluid pooling within the dependent pouch of Douglas.

catheter if need be. Unless the abscess is superficial or so large that it displaces adjacent and overlying bowel loops, the transabdominal route is limited. If suitable, the trocar technique of catheter placement can be used. Should there be concerns about the proximity of adjacent organs, vessels, or nerves, or if the abscess is small, the Seldinger technique should be employed (**Fig. 4**A,B).

Minimal or no sedation is required for this method, because local anesthetic instilled into the skin and subcutaneous track of the proposed catheter route is adequate in adults. The transabdominal route allows use of a standard 3- to

5-MHz curvilinear probe and larger bore catheters (8–14F), which hasten the drainage time and are more suitable for abscesses with particularly viscous contents. Transabdominal catheters are also more easily secured to the skin of the abdomen and more comfortable for the patient following the advent of nonsuture adhesive dressings. An example of a retention adhesive dressing is shown in **Fig. 2**A.

Percutaneous: Transgluteal

This approach can be more widely applied than the transabdominal route because it enables access to the deeper parts of the pelvis, particularly posterior to the rectum and sigmoid colon. Nevertheless, it involves transgression of the large gluteal muscles and passage of the catheter close to the sciatic nerve as it passes out of the greater sciatic notch, making it a more precarious choice of route. Although traditionally used in conjunction with CT due to the potential problem posed by the sciatic nerve and gluteal vessels, this route has been successfully performed under ultrasound guidance.[5,6]

The patient is placed in the prone position and conscious sedation is administered. This sedation is normally more substantial (fentanyl and midazolam) than that employed for the transabdominal route because the procedure is deemed to be more painful. A rectal tube and urinary catheter are useful to reduce the distension of both structures, thereby optimizing the sonographic window and minimizing unwanted lateral displacement of the catheter. Bony landmarks should be established. The coccyx is palpated, and an entry point as close and caudal to this is identified using

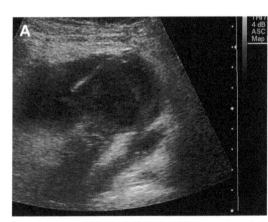
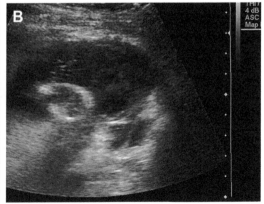

Fig. 4. (*A*) Transabdominal ultrasound image taken during a drainage using the Seldinger technique in a patient with an infected collection in close proximity to a pelvic transplant kidney. The needle can be seen correctly placed within the collection. (*B*) Subsequent view demonstrating catheter looped within the collection. Thick pus was aspirated and the catheter left on free drainage.

a standard 3- to 5-MHz curvilinear probe. By remaining close to the sacrococcygeal bones, damage to the neurovascular structures can be avoided. The Seldinger technique is used because a trocar does not allow the same degree of accuracy in a small field of access. The catheter (8–14F) is ideally placed at or below the level of the sacrospinous ligament, because the incidence of pain increases the more superior the point of access becomes. Once the catheter is deployed, it is usually fixed to the back of the thigh.

Advantages of this method include acceptability by those patients who refuse endocavitary drainage and reduction in the demand for CT time and consequently radiation exposure. A success rate of 81% has been quoted for CT-guided drainage,[7] with a similar outcome for ultrasound-guided drainage.[6] Most complications arise from inadvertent damage to the neurovascular bundle. This technique cannot be used in the obese because bony landmarks are difficult to palpate, and the subcutaneous fat layer becomes too deep to traverse safely.

Percutaneous: Transperineal

Originally developed for biopsy of the prostate,[8] the transperineal route has been adapted for use in the drainage of prostatic and deep pelvic (presacral) abscesses, particularly in patients who have undergone abdominoperineal resection and radiotherapy for rectal malignancy. Some patients prefer this route to an endocavitary one, providing an added option to consider when planning management.

The procedure requires the patient to be placed in the lithotomy position and again uses a standard linear or curvilinear probe. Conscious sedation (fentanyl and midazolam) is administered. The entry point for needle insertion should be as close to the midline as possible to avoid the pudendal nerves lying laterally within the ischiorectal fossae. The trocar technique has proved acceptable for this route of access, and many abscesses treated in this way are found to be small enough to resolve with aspiration alone. Alternatively, a small 8F catheter is commonly used. A distinct benefit of this approach is that transperineal drainage takes advantage of gravity, expediting abscess resolution. Larger catheters up to 12F can also be considered and secured by means of fixation to the skin of the perineum or thigh. Patients who have undergone radiotherapy tend to require protracted drainage times; therefore, anchorage of the catheter is important. Success rates as high as 100% have been described.[9,10] Complications are few and can be due to perineal neuralgia or

spontaneous displacement and expulsion of the catheter despite adequate fixation.

Endocavitary: Transvaginal and Transrectal

The transabdominal approach for drainage is used when possible, being more convenient for the patient and often requiring less sedation; however, if there is no safe route of access to the pelvis using this method, endocavitary routes of access provide an alternative (**Fig. 5**). Transvaginal and transrectal routes are similar and are discussed together.

Advocates of endocavitary drainage claim that, when compared with transgluteal drainage, endocavitary drainage is safer owing to avoidance of the major nerves and vessels as they pass through the greater sciatic foramen and less pain.[11] In addition, transgluteal drainage is often more expensive because it is a lengthier technique that usually requires CT guidance.

Transvaginal and transrectal routes are both effective and safe alternatives. Endocavitary probes now offer excellent visualization of deep-seated collections, including demonstrating detail regarding the internal architecture not possible with CT.

The route of choice will depend upon patient preference, radiologist experience, and the location of the collection and the accessibility by each route on preliminary imaging. The intervening rectum will limit access to more posterior or presacral collections via the transvaginal route. In addition, the transvaginal route is not recommended for drainage of collections high within the pelvis due to an increased risk of bowel, bladder, or vascular injury.

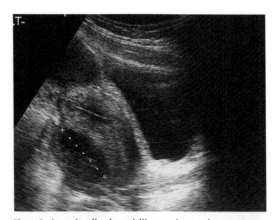

Fig. 5. Longitudinal midline view demonstrates a complex collection of mixed echogenicity within the pouch of Douglas. Transabdominal access is difficult, and the transvaginal route could provide a more suitable route of access.

The procedures are generally well tolerated, and patient acceptance of both transvaginal and transrectal catheters has been found to be high. Typically, a 7-MHz endocavitary probe is used. For transvaginal access, the patient lies supine with a wedge/cushion raising the patient's buttocks off the bed to allow probe manipulation. For transrectal access, the left lateral decubitus position is used.

There is no consensus within the literature regarding the need for local anesthesia or sedation. Some authorities describe the use of lidocaine to infiltrate either the posterior vaginal or rectal wall; some use local anesthesia only for vaginal procedures and not for rectal access; others routinely use both conscious sedation (eg, with fentanyl and midazolam) and local lidocaine, having found patient discomfort to be a problem during attempted penetration of the tough vaginal wall; and others have found local anesthesia entirely unnecessary.[11–14]

In the most commonly described technique, the endoprobe is covered with a sterile condom and a peelaway sheath attached to the side of the probe in the position that a standard needle guide could be sited. The sheath is fixed firmly in position using rubber bands (**Fig. 6**A,B). The collection is identified and the route assessed for the presence of large blood vessels or intervening structures that the catheter path will traverse. Usually, no incision is necessary for either needle or catheter insertion. Maintaining probe position, the trocar-mounted catheter can then be advanced into position through the peelaway sheath using continuous real-time visualization until the catheter tip is seen within the collection. The trocar is then removed, allowing pigtail formation (**Fig. 6**C,D). Once locked in position, the collection is aspirated to dryness.

As already described, an alternative to the trocar method is to use the Seldinger technique, but this method is more time-consuming and may be more painful, and there is an increased risk of kinking of wires and displacement during the maneuvers. Because of this risk, fluoroscopic screening is sometimes used to ensure that there is no loss of wire position. The Seldinger technique may be preferred in cases in which the collection is small or when close proximity to neurovascular structures or nearby organs would make a trocar

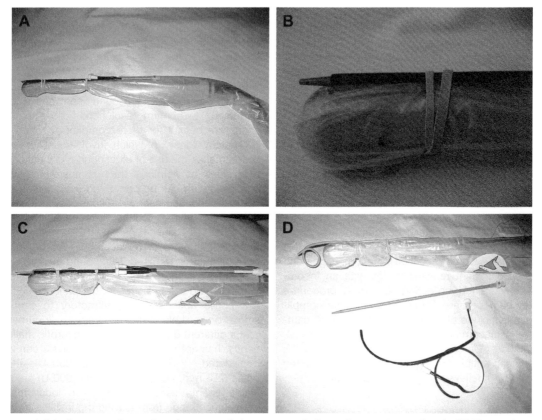

Fig. 6. (*A*) Probe set up for endocavitary use of the trocar technique via a peelaway sheath. (*B*) The peelaway sheath is securely attached to the probe using sterile elastic bands. (*C*) Using the trocar, the catheter can be placed into position through the sheath under direct ultrasound visualization. (*D*) Once in position, the catheter is locked.

technique unsafe, particularly when performing drainage via an endocavitary route. Some operators place a speculum and make a small nick in the cervix at the site of wire entry when using the Seldinger technique, because this may ease passage of the dilators. A nick within the coronal plane is said to reduce the risk of vascular injury. When aspiration only is required, the standard needle holder alone is clipped to the probe to guide needle placement.

For endocavitary access, catheter sizes of 8F are most commonly used, with smaller catheters being more easily sited. When collection contents are particularly viscous, the limit on catheter size of no greater than 10F can be a disadvantage of the endocavitary route.

Maintaining catheter position post deployment is more difficult with endocavitary drains than transabdominal ones, and most radiologists would recommend suturing the drain to the skin of the inner thigh.

Several authorities have reported excellent success rates with endocavitary catheter drainage, with rates comparable with those for transabdominal drainage.[12,15] Successful outcomes may also be achieved with aspiration alone, with the benefit of shorter procedure times and fewer complications, although repeated procedures may be necessary. For viscous fluid, the likelihood of success is greater with catheter drainage. Catheter drainage also allows for sinography when a fistula is suspected.

Transvaginal catheter drainage is safe, with a low rate of complications described in the literature, despite a theoretical risk of bleeding from the large blood vessels close to the vaginal vault. Failure to adequately drain thickened contents, such as can be found in infected hematomas, may result in the need for larger catheters to be placed via alternative routes, including transgluteal. Premature catheter dislodgement may occur (at rates between 4/17 and 4/40),[11,15] although this rarely has adverse effects on patient management. When a patient remains febrile with an incompletely drained collection, a repeat procedure may be necessary. Other reported minor complications include bladder transgression (2/40 catheter placements, treated conservatively), infection of a previously sterile collection (1/40, requiring antibiotic therapy), and catheter-related pain (1/40, relieved on catheter removal).[15]

CATHETER MANAGEMENT AND FOLLOW-UP

Once a catheter has been deployed and secured, the abscess or collection is aspirated to dryness, followed by irrigation with small aliquots (10–15 mL) of 0.9% normal saline, the repetition of which depends on the purulence and viscosity of the fluid drained. Care is taken to ensure that the volume of fluid instilled is less than that of the abscess contents to avoid increased intracavitary pressure and possible bacteremia. The catheter is then attached to a connecting tube and collection bag.

The cavity requires regular flushing with 5 to 10 mL of normal saline via the catheter anywhere between two and four times a day to reduce debris build up and consequent blockage. Daily rounds by the interventionalist to assess drainage are ideal but not always practical; hence, the input of the surgical team is important to ensure success. The catheter is left in situ until drainage has reduced to 10 to 15 mL/d and there is improvement in the patient's clinical condition. Sudden cessation of drainage should alert the clinician to blockage, whereas increased drainage volumes may indicate possible fistula formation. Monitoring of patient pyrexia is useful; any prolongation beyond 72 hours post catheter placement can indicate incomplete drainage or a coexistent source of sepsis. The white cell count is also valuable but generally has a slower response time. Should all parameters be favorable, the catheter can be withdrawn in both the ward and outpatient clinic setting. The decision to remove the catheter should involve the clinical team and the interventional radiologist.

Should any doubt exist with regards to drainage success, a repeat ultrasound can easily be performed to confirm resolution. Follow-up CT scans are helpful for more complex abscesses, particularly those in which involvement of the bowel makes the use of ultrasound more difficult. If a sinus or fistulous tract is suspected, an abscessogram can be performed using iodinated contrast and fluoroscopy. Occasionally, follow-up imaging reveals loculation or persistence of the abscess, and subsequent placement of multiple catheters or replacement with a larger bore catheter is required. Ultrasound guidance is far superior in these cases because its repeated use poses no safety issues for the patient.

If pelvic abscesses are refractory to simple single or multiple catheter drainage treatment and a different diagnosis, such as necrotic malignancy, has not become clear, fibrinolysis can be considered.[4,16] Streptokinase (120,000 U), alteplase (2–6 mg), and urokinase (500,000 U) are all viable agents used to breakdown loculations. Techniques range from leaving the instilled agent for 20 to 30 minutes before drainage and repeating the process several times a day to leaving the agent for 4 to 6 hours for a once-only treatment. The use of fibrinolytics is contraindicated in patients who have recently undergone surgery, are pregnant, or have had a hemorrhagic stroke.

SUMMARY

The role of interventional radiology in the treatment of pelvic abscesses and collections is increasing, helping to reduce the complexity of surgery or even eliminate the need for surgery at all. Although many imaging modalities and routes of access can be used, the increasing value of ultrasound guidance has been realized for even the most inaccessible of abscesses. Its benefits are clear in the pediatric patient, as well as proving to be cost-effective and versatile. Nevertheless, its limitations must be recognized, and a well-informed interventional radiologist can rapidly decide whether ultrasound-guided pelvic drainage is practical and safe.

REFERENCES

1. vanSonnenberg E, Wittich GR, Casola G, et al. Periappendiceal abscesses: percutaneous drainage. Radiology 1987;163(1):23–6.
2. Stabile BE, Puccio E, vanSonnenberg E, et al. Preoperative percutaneous drainage of diverticular abscesses. Am J Surg 1990;159(1):99–104.
3. Seldinger SI. Catheter replacement of the needle in percutaneous arteriography: a new technique. Acta Radiol 1953;39(5):368–76.
4. Gervais DA, Brown SD, Connolly SA, et al. Percutaneous imaging-guided abdominal and pelvic abscess drainage in children. Radiographics 2004; 24(3):737–54.
5. Harisinghani MG, Gervais DA, Hahn PF, et al. CT-guided transgluteal drainage of deep pelvic abscesses: indications, technique, procedure-related complications, and clinical outcome. Radiographics 2002;22(6):1353–67.
6. Walser E, Raza S, Hernandez A, et al. Sonographically guided transgluteal drainage of pelvic abscesses. AJR Am J Roentgenol 2003;181(2): 498–500.
7. Butch RJ, Mueller PR, Ferucci JT, et al. Drainage of pelvic abscesses through the greater sciatic foramen. Radiology 1986;158(2):487–91.
8. Rifkin MD, Kurtz AB, Goldberg BB. Sonographically guided transperineal prostatic biopsy: preliminary experience with a longitudinal linear-array transducer. AJR Am J Roentgenol 1983;140(4):745–7.
9. Sperling DC, Needleman L, Eschelman DJ, et al. Deep pelvic abscesses: transperineal US-guided drainage. Radiology 1998;208(1):111–5.
10. Barozzi L, Pavlica P, Menchi I, et al. Prostatic abscess: diagnosis and treatment. AJR Am J Roentgenol 1998;170(3):753–7.
11. Ryan RS, McGrath FP, Haslam PJ, et al. Ultrasound-guided endocavitary drainage of pelvic abscesses: technique, results and complications. Clin Radiol 2003;58:75–9.
12. Lucey B, Haslam P, Lee MJ. Pelvic abscess: technique and results of percutaneous drainage. Intervention 1999;3(1):3–12.
13. Maher MM, Gervais DA, Kalra MK, et al. The inaccessible or undrainable abscess: how to drain it. Radiographics 2004;24:717–35.
14. Nielson M Bachmann, Torp-Pederson S. Sonographically guided transrectal or transvaginal one-step catheter placement in deep pelvic and perirectal abscesses. AJR Am J Roentgenol 2004;183:1035–6.
15. Saokar A, Arellano R, Gervais D, et al. Transvaginal drainage of pelvic fluid collections: results, expectations, and experience. AJR Am J Roentgenol 2008; 191:1352–8.
16. Haaga JR, Nakamoto D, Stellato T, et al. Intracavitary urokinase for enhancement of percutaneous abscess drainage: phase II trial. AJR Am J Roentgenol 2000;174(6):1681–5.

Index

Note: Page numbers of article titles are in **boldface** type.

A

Abdominal interventions, **25–43**
   gallbladder, 30–31
   kidney. *See* Kidney.
   liver, 26–30
   lymph nodes, 37–40
   omentum, 34–36
   pancreas, 36–37
   peritoneum, 34–36
   radiofrequency ablation. *See* Radiofrequency
     ablation, of abdominal tumors.
   retroperitoneum, 31–34
   spleen, 37–40
   technology for, 25–26
Abdominal wall, fluid collections in, 40
Abscess
   hepatic, 29
   in radiofrequency ablation, 68
   pancreatic, 37
   pelvic, **73–81**
   pericholecystic, 31
   peritoneal, 34–36
   renal, 33–34
   splenic, 38
Acute tubular necrosis, 46
Air embolism, in lung biopsy, 23
Alcohol injection, with radiofrequency ablation, 65–67
Alport syndrome, kidney biopsy in, 51
Amebic abscess, liver, 29
Anesthesia
   for kidney biopsy, 47, 50
   for thyroid biopsy, 7
Anticoagulant therapy, kidney biopsy in, 47
Arteriovenous fistula, in kidney biopsy, 53–54
Ascites, drainage of, 34–36. *See also* Pelvic drainage.

B

Biopsy
   of abdominal wall, 40
   of gallbladder, 30–31
   of kidney, 31–34, **45–55**
   of liver, 26–30
   of lymph nodes, 37–40
   of omentum, 34–36
   of pancreas, 36–37
   of peripleural lung lesions, **17–24**
   of retroperitoneum, 34–36
   of spleen, 37–40
   of thyroid nodules, 5–9
   postthyroidectomy, 9–14

C

Carcinoma
   hepatocellular, 28
     radiofrequency ablation of. *See*
      Radiofrequency ablation, of abdominal
      tumors.
   thyroid, **1–16**
Catheter, for pelvic drainage, 80–81
Chemoembolization, with radiofrequency ablation, 67
Cholecystitis, 30–31
Cholecystostomy, 30–31
Coagulopathy, kidney biopsy in, 47
Color Doppler
   for abdominal interventions, 26–27
   for kidney biopsy, 32–33, 48
Comet-tail artifacts, in thyroid nodules, 4–5
Computed tomography, ultrasonography with, in lung
   biopsy, 23–24
Cyst(s)
   kidney, 34
   liver, 29

D

Diaphragm, radiofrequency ablation near, 68–69
Doxorubicin embolization, with radiofrequency
   ablation, 67
Drainage
   of abscess
     hepatic, 29
     renal, 34
     splenic, 38
   of pelvic fluid collections, **73–81**
   of peritoneal fluids, 34–36

E

Eggshell calcifications, in thyroid, 4
Electrocautery, with radiofrequency ablation, 67
Embolism, air, in lung biopsy, 23
Embolization, with radiofrequency ablation, 67
Endocavitary access, for pelvic drainage, 78–80
Enteric abscess, drainage of. *See* Pelvic drainage.
Ethanol injection, with radiofrequency ablation, 65–67

F

Fluid collections
   in abdominal wall, 40
   in kidney, 33
   in peritoneum, 34–36
   pelvic, **73–81**
Fusion imaging, for abdominal interventions, 26

doi:10.1016/S1556-858X(09)00027-9

ultrasound.theclinics.com

G

Gallbladder interventions, 30–31
Glomerulonephritis, 45–47, 51

H

Halo sign, in thyroid nodules, 5
Hematomas
    kidney, 33–34, 53
    pelvic, drainage of. *See* Pelvic drainage.
Hematuria
    after kidney biopsy, 46
    kidney biopsy for, 52–53
Hemorrhage
    in kidney biopsy, 53–54
    in lung biopsy, 23
    in radiofrequency ablation, 68
Hemothorax, in lung biopsy, 23
Hepatocellular carcinoma, 28
    radiofrequency ablation of. *See* Radiofrequency
        ablation, of abdominal tumors.
Hypertension, kidney biopsy in, 47

I

Interstitial nephritis, chronic, 46
Intestinal perforation, in radiofrequency ablation, 68

K

Kidney
    abscess of, 33–34
    biopsy of, 31–34, **45–55**
        complications of, 54
        contraindications for, 46–47
        indications for, 45–46
        monitoring after, 52–54
        patient setup for, 47
        prebiopsy scan for, 47–50
        procedure for, 50–51
        purpose of, 45
        specimen adequacy in, 51–52
    fluid collections in, 33
    solitary, 47
    tumors of, radiofrequency ablation of. *See*
        Radiofrequency ablation, of abdominal tumors.
    urinoma of, 33–34

L

Liver lesions, 26–30
    abscesses, 29
    biopsy of, 27–28
    cysts, 29
    metastatic, 28–30

radiofrequency ablation of. *See* Radiofrequency
    ablation, of abdominal tumors.
Lumpectomy, in abdominal wall, 40
Lung lesions, peripleural, **17–24**
Lymph nodes
    biopsy of
        in abdomen, 39–40
        in thyroid carcinoma, 9–14
    interventions for, 37–40
Lymphoceles
    kidney, 33–34
    pelvic, 36
        drainage of. *See* Pelvic drainage.
Lymphomas, of kidney, 34

M

Metastasis, to liver, 28–30, 67

N

Nephritis, chronic interstitial, 46
Nephrotic syndrome, 45

O

Omentum, interventions for, 34–36

P

Pancreas, biopsy of, 36–37
Pancreatitis, 37
Papillary carcinoma, thyroid, **1–16**
Paracentesis, 34–36
Pediatric patients
    kidney biopsy in, 45
    pelvic drainage in, 74
Pelvic drainage, **73–81**
    anatomic considerations in, 74–75
    catheter management in, 80–81
    contraindications for, 73–74
    endocavitary access for, 78–80
    indications for, 73
    patient preparation for, 75–76
    percutaneous access for, 76–78
    Seldinger technique for, 74, 79–80
    transabdominal access for, 76–77
    transgluteal access for, 77–78
    transperineal access for, 78
    transrectal access for, 78–80
    transvaginal access for, 78–80
    rocar technique for, 74, 79
Pericardium, radiofrequency ablation near,
    68–69
Peripleural lung lesions, **17–24**
Peritoneum, interventions for, 34–36

Peritonitis, spontaneous bacterial, 34–36
Pneumothorax
    in lung biopsy, 23
    in spleen biopsy, 38
Postthyroidectomy biopsy, 9–14
Pregnancy, kidney biopsy in, 47
Prostatic abscess, drainage of. See Pelvic drainage.
Proteinuria, 45–46
Pyogenic abscess, liver, 29
Pyuria, 46

R

Radiofrequency ablation, of abdominal tumors,
    57–71
    complications of, 68
    difficult regions in, 68–70
    electrocautery in, 67
    embolization with, 67
    ethanol injection with, 65–67
    history of, 57–58
    methods for, 65–67
    postablative management in, 67–68
    protocols for, 58–65
Rejection, after kidney transplantation, 46
Retroperitoneum, biopsy of, 31–34
Reverberation artifacts, in thyroid nodules, 4–5

S

Sclerotherapy
    for kidney cysts, 34
    for kidney lymphoceles, 33
Sedation
    for kidney biopsy, 47–48
    for pelvic drainage, 76
Seldinger technique, for pelvic drainage, 74,
    79–80
Seromas, kidney, 33–34
Sliding echogenic lung sign, in liver biopsy, 27

Spleen
    abscess of, 38
    interventions for, 37–40

T

Thyroid carcinoma, **1–16**
    anatomic considerations in, 2–3
    biopsy of, 5–9
    classification of, 3
    discovery of, 3
    thyroidectomy for, evaluation after, 9–14
    unrelated materials in, 3–4
    versus benign nodules, 4–5
Thyroid nodules
    benign versus malignant, 4–5
    classification of, 3
    incidence of, 3
    types of, 3–5
    unrelated materials in, 3–4
Thyroidectomy, biopsy after, 9–14
Transabdominal access, for pelvic drainage, 76–77
Transgluteal access, for pelvic drainage, 77–78
Transjugular approach, to liver lesions, 27
Transperineal access, for pelvic drainage, 78
Transplantation
    kidney, biopsy in, 32–33, 46, 50–53
    pancreas, biopsy in, 36–37
Transrectal access, for pelvic drainage, 78–80
Transvaginal access, for pelvic drainage, 78–80
Trocar technique, for pelvic drainage, 74, 79
Tubo-ovarian abscess, drainage of. See Pelvic
    drainage.

U

Ureteral injury, in radiofrequency ablation, 70
Urinary tract obstruction, kidney failure in, 46
Urinomas, 33–34

X

Xanthogranulomatous cholecystitis, 30–31

Printed and bound by CPI Group (UK) Ltd, Croydon, CR0 4YY

03/10/2024

01040362-0006